Mariani Foundation Paediatric Neurology Series
Editorial Board

Giuliano Avanzini, Milan, Italy
Philippe Evrard, Paris, France
Raoul Hennekam, Amsterdam, The Netherlands
Eugenio Mercuri, Rome, Italy
Fabio Sereni, Milan, Italy
Lawrence Wrabetz, Buffalo, NY, USA

Fondazione Pierfranco e Luisa Mariani
Viale Bianca Maria 28
20129 Milan, Italy

Telephone: +39 02 795458
Fax: +39 02 76009582
e-mail: publications@fondazione-mariani.org
www.fondazione-mariani.org

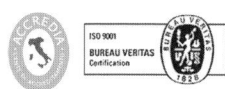

Fondazione con SGQ certificato

Cognitive and Behavioural Neurology in Developmental Age

Edited by

Daria Riva and Sara Bulgheroni

Mariani Foundation Paediatric Neurology Series: 28
Series Founder: Maria Majno
Associate Editor: Valeria Basilico

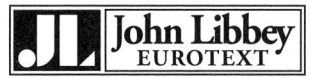

ISSN: 0969-0301
ISBN: 978-2-7420-1420-0

Cover design: Scriptoria (flower). Abstract image elaboration by Costanza Magnocavallo.

Technical and language editor: Oliver Gubbay.

Published by

Éditions John Libbey Eurotext
127, avenue de la République, 92120 Montrouge, France
Tel.: +33 (0)1 46 73 06 60
Fax: +33 (0)1 40 84 09 99
e-mail: contact@jle.com
www.jle.com

© 2015 John Libbey Eurotext. All rights reserved.

Unauthorized duplication contravenes applicable laws.

It is prohibited to reproduce this work or any part of it without authorization of the publisher or of the Centre Français d'Exploitation du Droit de Copie (CFC), 20, rue des Grands Augustins, 75006 Paris, France.

Contents

Chapter 1	The effect of brain lesions/disease on cognition: location/type and treatment *Daria Riva*	1

Epilepsy and headache

Chapter 2	Possible pathogenetic mechanisms of epileptic encephalopathies and implications for associated cognitive disorders *Silvana Franceschetti*	9
Chapter 3	Cognitive development in Dravet syndrome *Francesca Ragona, Mara Patrini and Tiziana Granata*	13
Chapter 4	The neuropsychological profile of childhood focal idiopathic epilepsy syndromes *Chiara Vago, Sara Bulgheroni, Silvia Esposito, Arianna Usilla and Daria Riva*	21
Chapter 5	Lesional epilepsies in childhood: neuropsychological and psychopathological aspects *Valentina Sibilia and Renzo Guerrini*	33
Chapter 6	Cognitive and behavioural aspects of headache in children and adolescents *Umberto Balottin, Matteo Chiappedi, Federica Galli, Sara Gianfelice and Cristiano Termine*	41

Malformations and tumours

Chapter 7	Spina bifida: brain and neurobehavioural outcomes *Jack M. Fletcher, Jennifer J. Juranek and Maureen Dennis*	49
Chapter 8	Neurocognitive, neuropsychological, and neurovisual development in single-suture craniosynostoses *Daniela Chieffo and Luca Massimi*	59

Chapter 9	Cognitive and behavioural outcome in children with posterior fossa malformations *Sara Bulgheroni, Fabiana Cazzaniga, Michela Bonalumi and Daria Riva*	69
Chapter 10	Brain tumours: how the location of the lesion and treatments affect cognitive function *Daria Riva, Silvia Esposito, Fabiana Cazzaniga and Sara Bulgheroni*	79
Chapter 11	Paediatric anaesthetic and cognitive neurotoxicity *Lena S. Sun*	85

Neurodevelopmental disorders

Chapter 12	Cognitive and behavioural phenotype in intellectual disability *Stefano Vicari, Paolo Alfieri and Deny Menghini*	99
Chapter 13	High-functioning autism spectrum disorders: focus on neuropsychological profiling *Antonio Narzisi, Filippo Muratori and Cosimo Urgesi*	109

Cerebral palsy

Chapter 14	Cognitive and language development in children with early focal brain lesions *Anna Maria Chilosi, Paola Brovedani, Sara Lenzi, Paola Cristofani and Paola Cipriani*	117
Chapter 15	Neuropsychological profiles in children with spastic diplegia with particular attention to visuo-cognitive abilities *Serena Micheletti, Jessica Galli and Elisa Fazzi*	127

Progressive neurological diseases

Chapter 16	Cognition and psychopathology in movement disorders in children *Nardo Nardocci and Mara Patrini*	139
Chapter 17	Lysosomal storage disorders *Rita Barone and Rossella Parini*	147
Chapter 18	Cognitive impairment in paediatric multiple sclerosis *Angelo Ghezzi*	167

Chapter 1

The effect of brain lesions/disease on cognition: location/type and treatment

Daria Riva

*Developmental Neurology Division, Fondazione IRCCS Istituto Neurologico 'C. Besta',
via Celoria 11, 20133 Milan, Italy*
Daria.Riva@istituto-besta.it

This introduction aims to outline the theoretical framework in which neuropsychological disorders, secondary to or associated with various types of diseases, locations, and types of brain lesions and their treatments, can be considered and examined. Higher psychic functions include a wide array of cognitive-behavioural functions that represent the final product of integrated processes of complex and widely distributed networks, made up of associative connections linking cortical areas that are highly or less highly specialized; the headquarters of sensory and motor elaborations which work together synchronously in a highly connected system. These widely distributed networks process the complexity and articulation of the language system, the visual-spatial capacity, and all other general abilities of the superior order (Riva, 2011).

The connectivity between brain areas is guaranteed by anatomical and functional connections. Structural anatomical connectivity is produced by a wide range of fibres, the classification of which, first made by Theodor Meynert in 1872 (Meynert, 1872), differentiates between associative and commissural projections. The projection pathways are: the corticobulbar tract, the corticospinal tract, the thalamo-cortical pathway and vice-versa, and the fornix pathway. There are also the commissural fibres, of which the corpus callosum is the most representative connecting system between the two hemispheres. There are, finally, associative fibres which are intra-hemispheric and connect associative areas of the same hemisphere.

The intra-hemispheric and commissural tracts thus compose the brain's structural and anatomical connectivity, that is, the discrete pathways that directly connect distant regions and territories. There is also a functional connectivity among brain regions that share functional properties. It can be defined, more specifically, as the spatial temporal correlation between neurophysiological and neuropsychological events that are spatially remote, but crucial to task-relevant processing. Functional connectivity, which can be analyzed using neurophysiological and direct functional brain imaging tools, has provided extraordinary information regarding brain function as well as, obviously, anatomical function, as it permits us to study *in vivo* human mental function and activity.

Knowledge about the brain's architecture is based on information furnished by different disciplines, including mathematical models known as Graph Theory (He & Evans, 2010) and advanced neuroimaging technologies, such as resting state functional magnetic resonance imaging. The latter method has made it possible to study the activation of specific brain areas even when the subject being examined is not engaged in an active task; it is also possible to investigate individuals with severe intellectual disability who are unable to carry out predetermined tasks.

According to mathematical models, instead, a network is usually made up of a clustering of more or less specialized areas which are connected to one another and, at the same time, to distant structures. The Graph Theory states that there are Small Worlds that are independent, although linked together by powerful internal connections, which do not work as a psychotic isolated system, but through in-between and distant connections with other Small Worlds. Functional connectivity is thus made up of hubs of greater or lesser complexity, convergences, divergences, feedback systems, switchboards, *etc.* which participate in the brain's extraordinarily complex processing system (Gerloff & Hallett, 2010).

Several important studies have made it possible to identify four functional networks, consistently found to be operative in healthy subjects: the visual, the sensorimotor, the basal ganglia (or basal nuclei), and *the Default Mode Network* (DMN). The latter is activated during passive mental no-task states (Buckner, 2012; Lee *et al.*, 2012; Moussa *et al.*, 2012).

The DMN operates in the morning when one is in a half-asleep state in which our minds are engaged in non-directed thinking; daydreaming, remembering, planning out everyday activities, linking memories and images, and planning freely without any definite logic. The DMN involves specific brain structures which include regions linked to episodic memory, those correlated to subjective visceral sensations processed in the precuneus, and to those processed by the inferior parietal lobes, an integrative area of fundamental importance. The organization of functional connections is not operative at an early age; the child's brain connects hubs and nodes in a unimodal processing system and the adult's brain connects areas within the confines of a multimodal one (integrative associative areas). There is thus a development over time; the infant has primary sensorimotor areas which are accessed by a single type of afference where it becomes integrated and, as the child develops, brain areas integrate different afferences. It can be said that between 7 and 9 years of age, the brain's architecture is similar to the Small-World type found in adults (Fransson *et al.*, 2010).

Brain architecture and function reflect a system in which some regions are more or less specialized while others are integrative and linked to one another by pathways. A lesion, be it malformative, tumoural, vascular, degenerative, or demyelinating, that damages one of the components of the system, causes a disconnection which fragments the integration process. If a lesion damages a hub or heteromodal (integrative) area, the impairment will be more significant with respect to secondary effects that are caused by nodal lesions. Any brain area is responsible for a part of the perfection of the final processing product. It is thus pointless to distinguish between eloquent and non-eloquent brain areas; it is instead important to distinguish between crucial, extremely complex areas, that might not be very vicarious, and less critical areas. The specialization of brain areas can be studied using various methodologies, such as morphological and functional MRI, combined positron emission tomography (PET), SPECT, *etc.*, while bundles of fibre tracts can be analyzed using diffusion tensor imaging (DTI) tractography, which allows us to analyze connectivity *in vivo*.

There is another added value to the disconnection paradigm; it is possible to uncover how lesions that are distant, for example, from language centres, can nevertheless provoke language disorders and to explain some neuropsychological syndromes that have been incomprehensible until now.

The model outlined by Catani and Ffytche in *Brain* in 2005 allows for the fact that brain disorders, and thus altered cognitive function or behavioural phenotypes, can be caused by topological mechanisms, that is, by the lesion's location or by odological mechanisms linked to disorders of the connecting system, or by both. This model provides insights into the neurological pathology even during developmental stages.

Studies focusing on the arcuate fasciculus can be used to exemplify *in vivo* investigations concerning connections between brain areas. The arcuate fasciculus connects Broca's area with Wernicke's area. The syndrome caused by a lesion to the fasciculus is characterized by language disorders; affected individuals are able to produce and understand words but not able to repeat them. The tractography studies revealed that the small tract of the arcuate fasciculus is actually made up of a pathway which directly connects Wernicke's area to Broca's area and of an indirect parallel pathway, of which nothing was previously known, composed of an anterior segment connecting Broca's area to the inferior parietal cortex, a powerful integrative area, and a posterior segment connecting Geschwind's with Wernicke's territories (Catani & Ffytche, 2005). This discovery made it possible to explain Geschwind's aphasic syndrome (named in honour of Geschwind, who first defined the disconnection syndrome). Patients with this syndrome are able to repeat words but have a limited verbal fluency and a lower verbal comprehension capacity.

The role of the second pathway between Broca's and Wernicke's areas is also extremely important for the acquisition of language; at the same time, it explains why children are able to repeat strings of sounds that have a semantic meaning (although they do not understand its meaning). In addition, it permits us to study reciprocal information, *i.e.* the bundles of connecting fibres are always bidirectional which means that the information travels from Wernicke's to Broca's area, but also from Broca's to Wernicke's area, both with regard to comprehension and verbal production (Riva, 2011).

Furthermore, another important issue is that the white matter and the cortical regions influence one another at the time of their maturation. If the connection system is altered, information arrives altered with a distorted pathological formation on the cortex; vice versa, a cortical region that is primitively pathological will have altered efferent connections and thus will have a deformed formative action on the connecting systems (Mesulam, 1990).

Even some neurodevelopmental disorders such as autism, with or without intellectual disability, can be explained by alterations in connections and regions. Autism is considered a prevalently pathogenetic disorder characterized by altered connectivity in which integrative areas are connected in an incomplete, pathological way due to faulty long connections; the short connections operating within a Small World appear, instead, to be so intensified that even high-functioning islands have been demonstrated. The fMRI studies have also confirmed that long connections are altered (Deshpande *et al.*, 2013).

In two recent studies, we examined autistic children with intellectual disability and found volume anomalies in some brain areas, including the basal forebrain, the cerebellum, and the mirror neuron system (Riva *et al.*, 2011, 2013). As a consequence, we expect to find that the connections between these areas are altered.

Even intellectual disability caused by genetic mutation has a place within this theoretical framework. Intellectual disability and anatomy are linked, and we can exemplify the correlation between the brain and phenotype by considering that a gene may code for a protein that enters and structurally takes part in cerebral circuits that process specific functions. If genetic mutations code for the absence of a protein or for an altered protein, the processing relative to the circuit(s) it is a part of will be altered, producing specific functional impairment and subsequently a distinct cognitive/behavioural phenotype for that mutation.

The neuroanatomical phenotype can become clearly evident on MRI, as in the case of Joubert's syndrome, of which the "molar tooth sign" (with deepened interpeduncular fossa and horizontalised, thickened and elongated superior cerebella peduncles) is pathognomonic (Maria et al., 1997). In other cases, the neuroanatomical phenotype is not so evident and must be detected using functional and advanced methodologies. We can use the example of the Fragile X syndrome to develop the concept that a malfunctioning or unexpressed protein in some brain regions processing a certain function can lead to a typical phenotype. This genetic condition, caused by a mutation of the *FMR1* gene due to the expansion of an unstable trinucleotide in the region of the gene, codes for a protein (the fragile X Mental Retardation Protein) expressed in many brain structures. The phenotype is characterized by learning disabilities of varying degrees which are generally more severe in males. The level of intellectual disability appears to be linked, according to a study of 144 families, to the quantity of FMRP protein. However, the most salient dissociation is that between verbal and visual perception abilities, to the detriment of the latter, with dysexecutive central syndrome and frequent autistic-like behaviour.

The FMRP protein in normal subjects is powerfully expressed in the magnocellular layers of the lateral geniculate nucleus, which is an integral part of the complex extrastriate visual areas of the dorsal stream dedicated to visual processing. Visual processing uses two basic pathways (besides the occipital striate cortex), the so-called visual extra-striate pathways. The ventral stream, which travels from the occipital lobes to the inferior temporal regions, is important for the analysis of characteristics regarding the form and colour of an object, while the dorsal pathway, which travels from the lateral geniculate body to the occipital lobes and then on to the parietal lobe, elaborates the spatial attributes of stimuli. In mutated FRAX subjects, this protein is either not expressed or expressed in an insufficient quantity; the outcome is that the extrastriate dorsal parietal circuit, which the geniculate body is a part of, is unable to adequately carry out visual tasks (Kaufmann et al., 1999).

Reiss and collaborators extensively studied the Fragile X syndrome, particularly in children younger than three compared with typically developing control subjects matched for age and sex (Gothelf et al., 2008). Utilizing volumetric, voxel-based, and surface-based modelling approaches, they found that abnormal development of specific brain regions characterizes a neuroanatomical phenotype associated with fragile X syndrome and may mediate the effects of *FMR1* gene mutations on the cognitive and behavioural features of the disorder. Further analyzes carried out by manually tracing the various structures confirmed the result that the most altered anatomical structure was both the left and right caudate which correlated with the lowest level of protein expression and with some scores of the autism scale and of the stereotypes (Gothelf et al., 2008).

Since a region is not independent of the connections that reach it, in the same way, the connections are not independent of the regions from which they originate or to where they are directed, and this results in a constant, reciprocal remodelling. Another study of the Fragile X syndrome used the tractography approach to show that the connections of the striate, of which the caudate is a part, and the frontal cortex were altered with a greater number and density of fibres with respect to those in normal or IQ-matched children (Haas *et al.*, 2009).

This means that abnormalities of the cortical regions and their connections in children over three confirm that there is an early genetic influence which selectively conditions brain architecture, giving rise to a typical anatomical phenotype and thus to an equally typical behavioural phenotype, which are correlated (Hoeft *et al.*, 2007).

Whenever the behavioural cognitive functions of a child with a neurological disorder are being studied, the treatments being utilized must always be taken into consideration. Differentiating between the effects of a primitive pathology and those of therapeutic medications is difficult and is an intuitively artificial process. Various types of treatment, be they surgical, radio or chemotherapeutic interventions, can cause important white matter structural alterations (see Riva's chapter on tumours in this book). As epilepsy is often associated with many neurological diseases, it is important to remember that antiepileptic drugs act at various levels and nearly all provoke cognitive disturbances (Ijff & Aldenkamp, 2013).

There are also some rehabilitative treatments that can even increase gene expression which controls neuronal plasticity. These findings confirm the importance of rehabilitation and underline the significance and potential of a discipline that has until only recently been markedly neglected. As demonstrated by the study of Maffei published in *Neuron* in 2007 (Pizzorusso *et al.*, 2007) and the one by Fischer published in the same year in *Nature* (Fischer *et al.*, 2007), the environmental enrichment, which is not necessarily synonymous with rehabilitation, but corresponds essentially to a caring approach or cognitive, social and physical stimulation, appears to trigger an epigenetic mechanism that can even alter the characteristics of some genes, which control plasticity. These genes are conditioned, in particular, in two specific brain regions, the hippocampus and neocortex, with a consequent increase in learning capacity and access to long-term memory. A group of investigators in Pisa recently reported that preterm infants who were given a massage showed an acceleration in visual evoked potentials and changes in electroencephalography (EEG) activity (Guzzetta *et al.*, 2009).

Conclusion

This chapter has outlined the theoretical framework in which the disorders described in this book are placed. The brain is a complex dynamic system formed by functionally interconnected regions; this has been demonstrated by clinical and lesion studies, and now by new neuroimaging techniques which have permitted us to study *in vivo* the specialization of regions and their connections, and to better understand clinical pictures which would otherwise be incomprehensible. A discrete lesion (tumour, stroke, or malformation) localized in specialized regions provokes specific deficits; lesions of hubs provoke more serious damage and white matter lesions provoke an important array of disabilities, including neurodevelopmental disorders. Various kinds of treatment/rehabilitation can modify cognitive behaviour, and environmental enrichment is known to increase cortical plasticity.

Conflicts of interest: none.

References

Buckner, R.L. (2012): The serendipitous discovery of the brain's default network. *Neuroimage* **62,** 1137–1145.

Catani, M. & Ffytche, D.H. (2005): The rises and falls of disconnection syndromes. *Brain* **128,** 2224–2239.

Deshpande, G., Libero, L.E., Sreenivasan, K.R., Deshpande, H.D. & Kana, R.K. (2013): Identification of neural connectivity signatures of autism using machine learning. *Front. Hum. Neurosci.* **7,** 670.

Fransson, P., Aden U., Blennow, M. & Lagercrantz, H. (2010): The functional architecture of the infant brain as revealed by resting-state fMRI. *Cereb. Cortex* **21,** 145–154.

Fischer, A., Sananbenesi, F., Wang, X., Dobbin, M. & Tsai, L.H. (2007): Recovery of learning and memory is associated with chromatin remodelling. *Nature* **447,** 178–182.

Gerloff, C. & Hallett, M. (2010): Big news from small world networks after stroke. *Brain* **133,** 952–955.

Gothelf, D., Furfaro, J.A., Hoeft, F., et al. (2008): Neuroanatomy of fragile X syndrome is associated with aberrant behavior and the fragile X mental retardation protein (FMRP). *Ann. Neurol.* **63,** 40–51.

Guzzetta, A., Baldini S., Bancale, A., et al. (2009): Massage accelerates brain development and the maturation of visual function. *J. Neurosci.* **29,** 6042–6051.

Haas, B.W., Barnea-Goraly, N., Lightbody, A.A., et al. (2009): Early white-matter abnormalities of the ventral frontostriatal pathway in fragile X syndrome. *Dev. Med. Child Neurol.* **51,** 593–599.

He, Y. & Evans, A. (2010): Graph theoretical modeling of brain connectivity. *Curr. Opin. Neurol.* **23,** 341–350.

Hoeft, F., Hernandez, A., Parthasarathy, S., Watson, C.L., Hall, S.S. & Reiss, A.L. (2007): Fronto-striatal dysfunction and potential compensatory mechanisms in male adolescents with fragile X syndrome. *Hum. Brain Mapp.* **28,** 543–554.

Ijff, D.M. & Aldenkamp, A.P. (2013): Cognitive side effects of antiepileptic drugs in children. *Handb. Clin. Neurol.* **111,** 707–718.

Kaufmann, W.E., Abrams, M.T., Chen, W. & Reiss, A.L. (1999): Genotype, molecular phenotype, and cognitive phenotype: correlations in fragile X syndrome. *Am. J. Med. Genet.* **83,** 286–295.

Lee, M.H., Hacker, C.D., Snyder, A.Z., et al. (2012): Clustering of resting state networks. *PLoS One* **7,** e40370.

Maria, B.L., Hoang, K.B., Tusa, R.J., et al. (1997): « Joubert syndrome » revisited: key ocular motor signs with magnetic resonance imaging correlation. *J. Child Neurol.* **12,** 423–430.

Mesulam, M.M. (1990): Large-scale neurocognitive networks and distributed processing for attention, language, and memory. *Ann. Neurol.* **28,** 597–613.

Meynert, T. (1872): Vom Gehirn der Saugetiere. In: *Handbuch der lehre von den geweben des menschen und tiere,* ed. S. Stricker, pp 694–808. Leipzig: Engelmann.

Moussa, M.N., Steen, M.R., Laurienti, P.J. & Hayasaka, S. (2012): Consistency of network modules in resting-state fMRI connectome data. *Plos One* **7,** e44428.

Pizzorusso, T., Berardi, N. & Maffei, L. (2007): A richness that cures. *Neuron* **54,** 508–510.

Riva, D. (2011): Higher cognitive function processing in developmental age: specialized areas, connections and distributed networks. In: *Brain Lesion Localization and Developmental Functions,* eds. D. Riva, C. Njiokiktjien, S. Bulgheroni, Mariani Foundation Paediatric Neurology Series, vol. 25, pp. 1–8. Montrouge: John Libbey.

Riva, D., Bulgheroni, S., Aquino, D., Di Salle, F., Savoiardo, M. & Erbetta, A. (2011): Basal forebrain involvement in low-functioning autistic children: a voxel-based morphometry study. *Am. J. Neuroradiol.* **32,** 1430–1435.

Riva, D., Annunziata, S., Contarino, V., Erbetta, A., Aquino, D. & Bulgheroni, S. (2013): Gray matter reduction in the vermis and CRUS-II is associated with social and interaction deficits in low-functioning children with autistic spectrum disorders: a VBM-DARTEL Study. *Cerebellum* **12,** 676–685.

Epilepsy and headache

Chapter 2

Possible pathogenetic mechanisms of epileptic encephalopathies and implications for associated cognitive disorders

Silvana Franceschetti

Dept. of Neurophysiopathology, Fondazione IRCCS Istituto Neurologico 'C. Besta', via Celoria 11, 20133 Milan, Italy
franceschetti@istituto-besta.it

Summary

In this chapter, some evidence regarding certain characteristics of epileptogenesis in the immature brain and the possible consequences affecting cognitive processes are summarised. Evidence suggests that, in experimental models, as in humans, the developing brain is prone to respond to epileptogenic events with more severe seizures. Moreover, the epileptogenic processes are concomitant with the physiological developmental phases, and the two evolving phenomena can negatively interact. In particular, the effect of the epileptogenic process on developmental plasticity can significantly disturb learning abilities.

In the rodent brain, major maturational events are prolonged after birth and involve both morphological and physiological aspects, moreover, most of the morphogenetic processes affecting cell bodies, dendrites, and axons also occur after birth. Cell bodies progressively enlarge and attain their final size by the end of the first month, while the volume of neuropil increases, mainly due to the growth of dendritic arborisation. Axonal proliferation and synapse formation occur at different rates in pyramidal and local circuit neurons, such that the axons of projection neurons begin to extend and form synapses before that of the axons of local circuit neurons.

Substantial changes in physiological properties occur concurrently with morphological development and involve both synaptic transmission and intrinsic membrane excitability.

In this chapter, we will summarize some evidence relating to the specific characteristics of epileptogenesis in the immature brain, as well as the possible perturbation affecting cognitive phenomena due to changes which occur within the window of time during early development, as a consequence of epileptogenic events.

Experimental studies support an increased susceptibility to seizures in the immature brain

Animal data support the assumption that the immature brain is intrinsically more susceptible to seizures, indeed epileptogenic manipulations performed in rodents (electrical stimuli, hypoxia, toxic agents or chemical convulsants) suggest that neonatal and juvenile animals have a lower seizure threshold and more severe seizures. This was demonstrated, in particular, for those chemical agents (kainate and pilocarpine) that induce an initial epileptic status and represent a model of temporal lobe epilepsy (characterized by spontaneous recurrent seizures) after a variable latent period (for a review, refer to Wong, 2005).

Immature neurotransmission is pro-epileptogenic: the special case of GABA

The developmental rearrangement of the neurotransmitters and receptors is a factor that may significantly predispose the immature brain to increased seizure susceptibility. go toward

All neurotransmitters are involved in post-natal maturational processes, but an extremely important factor appears to depend on the specific maturational profile of the main inhibitory neurotransmitter, gamma aminobutyric acid (GABA). In fact, GABA is present in the brain even before GABAergic synapses are formed and probably plays an early trophic function, influencing the differentiation and migration of neurons (for a recent review, refer to Nardou *et al.*, 2013). When GABA starts to exert a neurotransmitter effect, it behaves as an excitatory rather than an inhibitory neurotransmitter. This paradoxical effect derives from the specific distribution of chloride ions in the immature brain due to the presence of an immature form of the chloride membrane pump, which actively causes influx of chloride ions and results in an intracellular chloride concentration more than three times greater than that found in mature neurons. Because of this particular condition, GABA action results in a membrane depolarization that can lead to action potential generation.

Epileptogenesis and seizure-induced changes in cortical structures

Seizure-induced changes in cortical structures demonstrated in animal models (mainly rodents) have been commonly obtained after initial brain damage induced by different methods, most of which represent a model of the process leading to temporal lobe epilepsies. In theses studies, the epileptogenic process includes acute changes, immediately following the epileptogenic manipulation, with rapid alterations in ion channel kinetics and functional proteins, and activation of immediate early genes, followed by sub-acute changes occurring through a period of weeks, including transcriptional events, neuronal death, and activation of inflammatory events.

Chronic changes that follow over weeks to months include aberrant neurogenesis and axonal sprouting network reorganization, as well as gliosis. All these epileptogenic processes interact with physiological developmental processes and might contribute to differences in epileptogenesis between adult and developing brains (for a review, refer to Wong [2005] and Rakhade & Jensen [2009]).

Some of the experimental methods used in rodent studies to induce epileptic status (*e.g.* chemicals convulsants administered systemically or within specific brain structures) have a significant value in our understanding of the mechanisms of the progressive epileptogenic processes, but a doubtful relevance for a clinical point of view. However, important chronic changes have also been obtained with experimental manipulations, such as hypoxia or induced febrile seizures (Jensen *et al.*, 1992; Chang *et al.*, 2003), which more closely reproduce clinical situations.

In fact, the profile of changes induced by epileptogenic manipulation clearly differs in young animals compared to mature animals. Widespread evidence obtained from several animal models over many years (*e.g.* Cavalheiro *et al.*, 1987), indicates that, in immature animals, the lesional events following the early epileptogenic manipulation are minimal when compared with those induced in mature animals, even in the case of epileptic status or severe early seizures. Therefore, we should assume that subtle structural changes or specific functional rearrangements give rise to epileptogenesis and associated cognitive and behavioural dysfunctions in the absence of obvious brain damage (for a review, refer to Stafstrom, 2007).

Early seizures can alter either excitatory or inhibitory neurotransmitter receptor distribution, composition, and density, and neurotransmitter transporters (Zang *et al.*, 2004) can be altered by seizures occurring early during development, leading to a permanent state of hyperexcitability.

Distorted cell function and circuitry may interfere with cognitive development

A main issue concerning epilepsies in infancy relates to the interaction between seizures, epileptogenic processes, and development of cognitive functions. Human studies certainly suggest that seizures are damaging in infancy and childhood. In fact, children with early epilepsies often display neurocognitive deficits, which can be progressive and may correlate with seizure frequency. However, in humans, it is hard to distinguish between the effect of seizures and other factors, such as the underlying aetiology or the effect of antiepileptic drugs.

Animal models allow to better control these variables and reach a clearer picture of the mechanism involved in seizure-induced deficits. However, although the experimental evidence can explain some seizure effects, it cannot be assumed that this broadly relates to all human epilepsies.

Several lines of laboratory evidence demonstrate that seizures occurring early in infancy can result in permanent defects in learning ability (Lynch *et al.*, 2000; Sayin *et al.*, 2004; see Stafstrom, 2007 for a review) and various efforts have been made to identify the precise mechanism of such defective development. In fact, the recognition of the precise relationship between early seizures and learning deficits should make it feasible to establish corrective strategies.

Given that seizure-induced anatomical damage and neuronal cell death is minimal in very young rodents, epileptic events occurring at early ages are expected to negatively influence learning abilities through more subtle changes in the nervous system, such as abnormal neuronal connectivity and synaptic reorganization ('proutin'). For instance, the subunits of the AMPA subfamily of glutamate receptors can be permanently altered even after a single episode of neonatal seizures (Cornejo *et al.*, 2007). In addition, rats with neonatal seizures may undergo changes in modulating proteins involved in synaptic plasticity and this may represent a general model of negative effect of seizures on learning processes, even if the spectrum of potential interference is so large that it is not possible at present to identify a key strategy to counteract distorted plasticity.

Conflicts of interest: none.

References

Cavalheiro, E.A., Silva, D.F., Turski, W.A., Calderazzo-Filho, L.S., Bortolotto, Z.A. & Turski, L. (1987): The susceptibility of rats to pilocarpine-induced seizures is age-dependent. *Brain Res.* **465**, 43–58.

Chang, Y.C., Huang, A.M., Kuo, Y.M., Wang, S.T., Chang, Y.Y. & Huang, C.C. (2003): Febrile seizures impair memory and cAMP response-element binding protein activation. *Ann. Neurol.* **54**, 706–718.

Cornejo, B.J., Mesches, M.H., Coultrap, S., Browning, M.D., Timothy, A. & Benke, T.A. (2007): A single episode of neonatal seizures permanently alters glutamatergic synapses. *Ann. Neurol.* **61**, 411–426.

Jensen, F.E, Holmes, G.L, Lombroso, C.T., Blume, H.K. & Firkusny, I.R. (1992): Age-dependent changes in long-term seizure susceptibility and behavior after hypoxia in rats. *Epilepsia* **33**, 971–980.

Lynch, M., Sayin, U., Bownds, J., Janumpalli, S. & Sutula, T. (2000): Long-term consequences of early postnatal seizures on hippocampal learning and plasticity. *Eur. J. Neurosci.* **12**, 2252–2264.

Nardou, R., Ferrari, D.C. & Ben-Ari, Y. (2013): Mechanisms and effects of seizures in the immature brain. *Semin. Fetal. Neonatal. Med.* **18**, 175–184.

Rakhade, S.N. & Jensen, F.E. (2009): Epileptogenesis in the immature brain: emerging mechanisms. *Nat. Rev. Neurol.* **5**, 380–391.

Sayin, U., Sutula, T.P. & Stafstrom, C.E. (2004): Seizures in the developing brain cause adverse long-term effects on spatial learning and anxiety. *Epilepsia* **45**, 1539–1548.

Stafstrom, C.E. (2007): Neurobiological mechanisms of developmental epilepsy: translating experimental findings into clinical application. *Semin. Pediatr. Neurol.* **14**, 164–172.

Wong, M. (2005): Advances in the pathophysiology of developmental epilepsies. *Semin. Pediatr. Neurol.* **12**, 72–87.

Zhang, G., Raol, Y.S.H., Hsu, F-C. & Brooks-Kayal, A.R. (2004): Long-term alterations in glutamate receptor and transporter expression following early life seizures are associated with increased seizure susceptibility. *J. Neurochem.* **88**, 91–101.

Chapter 3

Cognitive development in Dravet syndrome

Francesca Ragona, Mara Patrini and Tiziana Granata

Paediatric Neurosciences Division, Fondazione IRCCS Istituto Neurologico 'C. Besta', via Celoria 11, 20133 Milan, Italy
francesca.ragona@istituto-besta.it

Summary

Dravet syndrome (DS) is an epileptic encephalopathy associated in most cases with *de novo* mutations of the *SCN1A* gene, which encodes the voltage-gated sodium channel Nav1.1. Febrile and afebrile, generalized and/or focal seizures appear during the first year of life in previously healthy children. In the following years, recurrent polymorphic seizures, stagnation of psychomotor development, and appearance of neurological signs enrich the clinical picture. Prognosis is unfavourable in most cases and seizures become drug-resistant; all patients exhibit motor deficits, moderate to severe cognitive impairment, and behaviour disorders. Developmental and behaviour disorders represent one of the most important invalidating clinical problems for the patients and their family and should be addressed as a crucial part of the comprehensive care for Dravet patients. Developmental delay has been historically considered to be the result of recurring seizures, hence the inclusion of DS among the epileptic encephalopathies. However, literature data and personal experience question this univocal correlation and suggest that DS encompasses different epileptic and cognitive phenotypes that probably result from different genetic and epigenetic factors. Epilepsy is probably one of the variables, together with pharmacological treatment, rehabilitation, and social and familial environment, which concur in determining the cognitive outcome.

Introduction

Dravet syndrome (DS), also termed Severe Myoclonic Epilepsy of Infancy (SMEI), is an epileptic syndrome, associated, in most cases with *de novo* mutations of the *SCN1A* gene, which encodes the voltage-gated sodium channel Nav1.1 (Claes *et al.*, 2001). The disease presents in the first year of life in an otherwise healthy child with febrile and afebrile, generalized and/or focal seizures. The disease course is characterized by slowing of psychomotor development, appearance of neurological signs, and recurrent polymorphic seizures in the form of focal, myoclonic, atypical absences, generalized or unilateral clonic and tonic-clonic (Dravet, 1978). EEG, which is usually normal at onset, will subsequently show generalized and focal discharges, photosensitivity, and slowing of background activity (Dalla Bernardina *et al.*, 1982; Dravet *et al.*, 2002). Prognosis is unfavourable in most cases and seizures become drug-resistant; all patients exhibit motor and cognitive impairment, usually moderate or severe. A less severe variant of DS, termed SMEI-borderline (SMEB), lacking

13

absences and myoclonus, has been described (Ogino *et al.*, 1988). Stagnation in psychomotor development is consistently reported and represents one of the key features of the disease, both in SMEI and in SMEB; starting from the second year of life, language progresses very slowly, ambulation becomes uncertain, and instability and attention deficits appear. Language and visuo-spatial skills are the first functions to be impaired, but in the following years, slowing of achievements involves all the neuropsychological areas.

Developmental delay has been historically considered to be the result of severe epilepsy, hence the inclusion of DS among epileptic encephalopathies (Engel, 2001). However, data from the literature and personal experience question a direct correlation between the course of epilepsy and cognitive outcome (Ragona *et al.*, 2008, 2010; Riva *et al.*, 2009) and suggest that the genetic defect also plays a pivotal role in neurobehavioural comorbidities.

Review of the topic

Despite the prominence of cognitive and behavioural disorders in DS, only a few studies have specifically dealt with this topic. The analysis of the literature is, moreover, hampered by the different methods employed to assess the cognitive functions in the different series of patients reported. Finally, genetic data are available only in the most recent literature. The first reported study focussing on the cognitive evolution in DS patients is that of Wolff and co-authors who studied a series of 20 children aged 11 months to 16 years. The cognitive evolution was assessed by the analysis of developmental milestones and by the Brunet-Lézine Developmental Scale; behaviour was assessed by means of observation during testing and free play. Cognitive development and behaviour were normal in all cases at disease onset; stagnation of psychomotor development became evident in all cases from the second year of life and resulted in a progressive decline of developmental quotient until the age of 4 years. All children displayed behavioural disturbances such as mood instability and hyperactivity. In 12 of the 20 cases, the longitudinal neuropsychological data were correlated to the following variables: personal and family history, neuroimaging, age at onset of epilepsy, seizure types, and frequency. The authors observed a correlation trend between the severity of intellectual disability and the high frequency of convulsive seizures (> 5 per month); based on this observation, the authors suggested that the frequency of convulsive seizures may constitute a major risk factor for intellectual disability, and that Dravet syndrome may be considered a true epileptic encephalopathy (Cassé-Perrot *et al.*, 2001; Wolff *et al.*, 2006). This report should be rewarded as the first to evaluate the potential role of epilepsy in determining cognitive evolution. Nonetheless, the conclusion of the authors must be considered cautiously because of the following limits: the correlation between epilepsy and cognitive course was available only for a small subset of patients; in no case was genetic analysis performed; and most importantly, the age of children at the last examination varied widely, ranging between 11 months and 12 years. Indeed, the three patients who performed better were among the youngest of the series (11, 21 and 28 months, respectively), thus the possibility of cognitive delay in later ages cannot be ruled out.

Caraballo and Fejerman (2006) evaluated the clinical records of 53 patients (mean age: 11 years; range: 4-14 years). The diagnosis was based on clinical criteria and no molecular studies were performed. Thirty-nine patients met the clinical diagnostic criteria of SMEI and 14 patients could be classified as SMEB as they never experienced myoclonias. All the patients were systematically evaluated by means of WPPSI tests which revealed, starting from the age of 2 years, cognitive delay in all cases. At the last examination, obtained between 4 and 14 years (mean age: 11 years), mental delay was mild in 34 per cent, moderate in 41.5 per cent, and

Chapter 3 Cognitive development in Dravet syndrome

severe in 26 per cent of the patients. Behaviour disturbances were also present in the large majority of patients, mainly defined as hyperactivity (85 per cent of patients); only two patients (3.5 per cent) were affected by autism. We obtained similar results in a series of 37 patients; mental deficits of various degrees were present in all the children evaluated after the age of six years. Twenty-three patients among the 37 had been evaluated longitudinally, for a mean period of 6.3 years, by serial standardized cognitive assessment (the Griffiths's or Wechsler scales according to the age and level of collaboration). By stratifying the patients according to age at last examination, it appears that the percentage of patients with severe intellectual disability increased with increasing age (Fig. 1). This apparent worsening reflects the arrest of cognitive development that took place in all cases up to the age of 5 years. Developmental quotient falls until the age of six and then remains stable; the observed decline in IQ scores in the following years is due to the rising discrepancy between the steady mental age and increasing chronological age. Moreover, as the patients grew up, the disability was worsened by behaviour disorders, evident in 21 patients, characterized by attention deficit, hyperactivity, and opposition. Only in four patients was the phenotype consistent with the diagnosis of generalized development disorder. This study confirms that cognitive decline became evident at the time of higher seizure frequency (the first 4-5 years of age), but also that patients with similar epileptic history may have different cognitive evolution. These observations suggest that both epilepsy and the channelopathy contribute in determining the final outcome (Ragona et al., 2008, 2010). Similar conclusions were reached by Riva and colleagues, who described the cognitive evolution of two children affected by DS, associated with *de novo SCN1A* truncating mutations. The longitudinal assessment was carried out by the same expert neuropsychologist, by means of the Griffiths Mental Developmental Scales, from 11 months to 7 years (Case 1) and from 23 months to 8 years (Case 2). In spite of the different course of their epileptic histories (Case 1 had frequent polymorphic seizures, including daily myoclonic jerks; Case 2 had rare tonic-clonic seizures with long seizure-free periods), the two patients experienced early mental malfunctioning and subsequent cognitive impairment. According to these data, the authors suggested that *SCN1A* mutations have a major role in mental impairment, suggesting

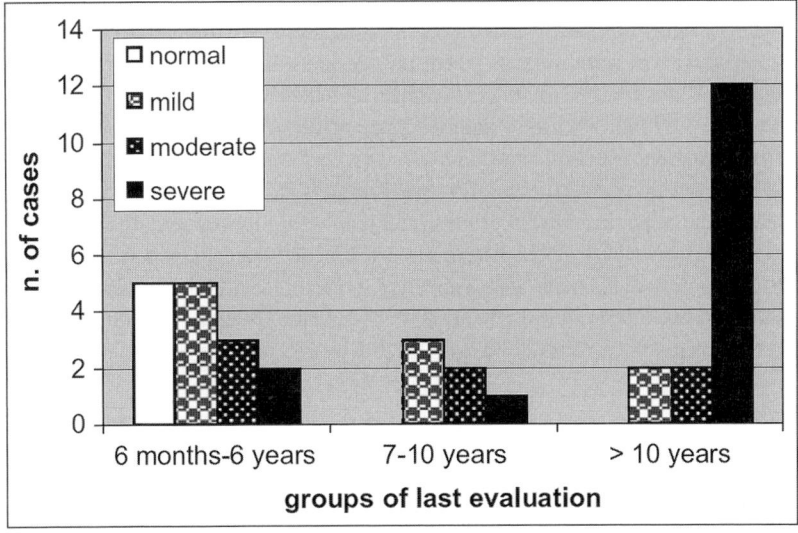

Fig. 1. Results of cognitive evaluation in the different age groups.

that the gene can be a candidate gene for intellectual disability (Riva *et al.*, 2009). The putative role of channelopathy in determining cognitive outcome was also discussed by Guzzetta and colleagues in a study aimed at describing the early neuropsychological evolution of five Dravet patients, one of whom had an *SCN1A* truncating mutation. Cognition and behaviour were evaluated by the Griffiths Scale and CBCL; visual function was tested through the evaluation of ocular motility, attention over distance, acuity, visual fields, fixation shift, and stereopsis. Four of the five patients had visual impairment at the first evaluation, which was performed within 2 years of life in four cases and at 30 months in one case; in all cases, the visual abnormalities preceded the cognitive decline. The only patient with normal visual function had normal cognitive profile at the end of follow-up (GQ of 94 at 51 months of age). The authors underlined the prognostic value of visual impairment and recommend to perform early and sequential assessments of visual function in all cases of DS (Chieffo *et al.*, 2011a). A role for the channelopathies in determining cerebellar dysfunction, responsible for specific neuropsychological deficits, has been advocated by the same group based on a study of nine DS patients (five of whom carried *SCN1A* mutations), classified as SMEB (five cases) or SMEI (four cases), which were compared to a control group which included nine patients with other epilepsies, matched by age and IQ. The authors found that DS patients had a specific pattern of cognitive defects, consistent with a 'cerebellar affective syndrome', characterized by deficits in the following areas: expressive language (with relatively spared comprehension), visual-spatial organization, executive functions, and behaviour (Chieffo *et al.*, 2011b; Battaglia *et al.*, 2013).

Data from an Italian collaborative longitudinal study

In an attempt to clarify the respective roles of epilepsy course and genetic alteration in determining the final cognitive outcome, an Italian multicentric study was started in 2006, based on a grant from the Mariani Foundation. This included both a retrospective and a prospective study; the latter is still in progress. In the retrospective study, we reviewed the clinical history and cognitive development of 26 patients, collected from five Italian centres, who met the following inclusion criteria: (1) clinical diagnostic criteria for Dravet syndrome; (2) screening for molecular analysis of the *SCN1A* gene; (3) clinical course clearly traceable on the basis of clinical charts and family diaries, particularly with regard to frequency and semiology of seizures; and (4) at least two standardized cognitive evaluations by the age of five, of which the first was performed within 1 year from the onset of seizures. The upper limit of assessment was set based on previous studies indicating that arrest of cognitive development occurred within the first years after seizure onset (Cassé-Perrot *et al.*, 2001; Ragona *et al.*, 2010). Each patient underwent serial standardized cognitive evaluation, by means of the Griffiths's Scale or Brunet Lezine and Wppsi, according to age and level of collaboration. The cognitive outcome was quantified as differential general quotient (dGQ) between 12 and 60 months. Statistical analysis correlated the dGQ with genotype and epilepsy course. The epilepsy course was reviewed with particular attention to age at onset of seizures, seizure types and mean frequency of convulsions, absences, myoclonic seizures, and to the number of prolonged seizures and status.

Epilepsy started at the mean age of 5.6 months. All the patients experienced prolonged convulsive seizures, whereas absences and myoclonus were reported in 17 cases. Cognitive outcome was poor in almost all patients (mean dGQ being 33 points), but with a decreased range varying from 6 to 77 points. Based on the statistical analysis of the whole series, correlations between cognitive outcome and genotype or epilepsy course were not identified. Nevertheless, based on the analysis of individual cognitive profiles, seven patients were identified with dGQ lower than 20 points: the main clinical characteristic in this subset of patients was the lack of early absences and myoclonus. These data suggest that DS encompasses different epileptic and cognitive phenotypes that probably result from different genetic and epigenetic factors. The epileptic phenotype appears to bear a prognostic value, as the early appearance of myoclonus and absences is associated with the worst cognitive outcome. (Ragona, 2011; Ragona et al., 2011). The prospective study is still ongoing. We are enrolling children aged less than 14 months who meet the following inclusion criteria: normal psychomotor development and no significant personal antecedents, onset of seizures in the first year of life in the form of at least two febrile convulsions, or afebrile convulsions, either prolonged (*i.e.* > 15 minutes) or unilateral or with localized onset and subsequent generalization.

All the enrolled children are undergoing *SCN1A* gene screening (sequencing and MLPA) and complete neuropsychological assessment based on the Griffiths Scale, Vineland Scale, and Child Behaviour Checklist, every six months from the onset of the disease.

This prospective study allows us to compare Dravet patients with a 'control group', which includes patients with simple febrile convulsions, focal cryptogenetic epilepsy, and other 'non-lesional' epilepsies. The preliminary results suggest that, from the second year of life, the Dravet patients have a GQ lower than that of the control group, regardless of the different aetiology of the control patients. Moreover, in DS patients, the frequency of seizures at the time of evaluation had a significant impact on the cognitive profiles; patients did better when tests were administered during seizure-free periods and did worst during periods of high seizure frequency. In the control group, the cognitive profiles appeared to be more consistent during the disease course.

Conclusions

Stagnation in psychomotor development, which becomes evident from the second year of life, represents one of the key features of DS. Over the following years, behaviour disorders, together with the progressive evidence of intellectual disability, become the most invalidating clinical problems for the patients and their families. Behavioural and cognitive problems are indeed reported to be one of the principal predictors of health-related quality of life in adult patients, independent of epilepsy-related problems (Brunklaus et al., 2011). The management of developmental disorders should therefore be considered as a crucial part of the comprehensive care for Dravet patients (Granata, 2011). A complete neuropsychological assessment which includes cognitive, behavioural, and adaptive evaluation should be performed as close as possible to seizure onset and repeated every six months, during the first four years of life, then annually. We suggest that the following standardized and repeatable tests should be applied in order to evaluate patients longitudinally: the Griffiths Mental Development Scales, Vineland Scale, Child Behaviour Checklist, behaviour observation, and specific assessment of attention, language, and visual skills. The serial assessments help to pinpoint the rising problems and plan ahead for appropriate treatment; cognitive rehabilitation by psychomotor and speech therapy. Moreover, the evaluation session is the setting where the family is helped to understand and accept the emerging difficulties, and where suggestions for upbringing are provided. As the patients grow up, behaviour disorders may become prominent and require behavioural and cognitive treatments, and, in selected cases, pharmacological treatment for hyperactivity, aggressiveness, and obsessive compulsive disorders. In our experience, the newly-diagnosed patients appear to have less severe cognitive impairment when compared to our previous series; this improvement might be related, not only to a more appropriate pharmacological treatment (avoidance of heavy drug load and avoidance of contraindicated drugs), but also to the more comprehensive care offered to newly-diagnosed patients. The pathogenesis of cognitive stagnation is not completely understood and the respective roles of epilepsy and genetic background in determining the cognitive outcome of patients with Dravet syndrome is still a matter for study. Developmental delay has been historically considered to be the result of recurring seizures, hence the inclusion of DS among epileptic encephalopathies. However, data from the literature and personal experience question a direct correlation between the course of epilepsy and cognitive outcome. It is conceivable that Dravet syndrome encompasses different epileptic and cognitive phenotypes that probably result from different genetic and epigenetic factors, and that epilepsy is just one of the variables that plays a role in cognitive development. Many other variables, such as pharmacological treatment, rehabilitation, and social and familial environment, probably concur in determining the overall outcome. Prospective analysis of large series of patients might allow us to identify correlations between epilepsy phenotype, genetic alteration, and cognitive outcome, and hopefully lead to improved care for patients with DS.

Acknowledgments: this work was supported by a grant from the Mariani Foundation (Milan, Italy).

Conflicts of interest: none.

References

Battaglia, D., Chieffo, D., Siracusano, R., *et al.* (2013): Cognitive decline in Dravet syndrome: is there a cerebellar role? *Epilepsy Res.* **106**, 211–221.

Brunklaus, A., Dorris, L. & Zuberi, S.M. (2011): Comorbidities and predictors of health-related quality of life in Dravet syndrome. *Epilepsia* **52**, 1476–1482.

Caraballo, R.H. & Fejerman, N. (2006): Dravet syndrome: a study of 53 patients. *Epilepsy Res.* **70**, 231–238.

Cassé-Perrot, C., Wolff, M. & Dravet, C. (2001): Neuropsychological aspects of severe myoclonic epilepsy in infancy. In: *Neuropsychology of Childhood Epilepsy*, eds. I. Jambaque, M. Lassonde & O. Dulac, pp. 131–140. New York: Kluver Academic/Plenum Publishers.

Chieffo, D., Ricci, D., Baranello, G., *et al.* (2011a): Early development in Dravet syndrome: visual function impairment precedes cognitive decline. *Epilepsy Res.* **93**, 73–79.

Chieffo, D., Battaglia, D., Lettori, D., *et al.* (2011b): Neuropsychological development in children with Dravet syndrome. *Epilepsy Res.* **95**, 86–93.

Claes, L., Del-Favero, J., Ceulemans, B., Lagae, L., Van Broeckhoven, C. & De Jonghe, P. (2001): De novo mutations in the sodium-channel gene *SCN1A* cause severe myoclonic epilepsy of infancy. *Am. J. Hum. Genet.* **68**, 1327–1332.

Dalla Bernardina, B., Capovilla, G. & Gattoni, M.B. (1982): Épilepsie myoclonique grave de la première année. *Rev. EEG Neurophysiol.* **12**, 21–25.

Dravet, C. (1978): Les épilepsies graves de l'enfant. *Vie. Méd.* **8**, 543–548.

Dravet, C., Bureau, M. & Oguni, H. (2002): Severe myoclonic epilepsy in infancy (Dravet Syndrome). In: *Epileptic Syndromes in Infancy, Childhood and Adolescence*, eds J. Roger, M. Bureau, C. Dravet, P. Jenton, C.A. Tassinari & P. Wolff, pp. 75–88. London: John Libbey.

Engel, J. Jr.; International League Against Epilepsy (ILAE). (2001): A proposed diagnostic scheme for people with epileptic seizures and with epilepsy: report of the ILAE task force on classification and terminology. *Epilepsia* **42**, 796–803.

Granata, T. (2011): Comprehensive care of children with Dravet syndrome. *Epilepsia* **52**, 90–94.

Ogino, T., Ohtsuka, Y., Amano, R., Yamatogi, Y. & Ohtahara, S. (1988): An investigation on the borderland of severe myoclonic epilepsy in infancy. *Jpn. J. Psychiatry Neurol.* **42**, 554–555.

Ragona, F. (2011): Cognitive development in children with Dravet Syndrome. *Epilepsia* **52**, 39–43.

Ragona, F., Offredi, F., Morbi, F., *et al.* (2008): Cognitive development in Dravet syndrome: a retrospective, multicentre study of twenty seven patients. In: *Abstracts from the 8th European Congress on Epileptology*, eds. M. Bialer & C. Elger, p. 69.

Ragona, F., Brazzo, D., De Giorgi, I., *et al.* (2010): Dravet syndrome: early clinical manifestations and cognitive outcome in 37 Italian patients. *Brain Dev.* **32,** 71–77.

Ragona, F., Granata, T., Dalla Bernardina, B., *et al.* (2011): Cognitive development in Dravet syndrome: a retrospective, multicenter study of 26 patients. *Epilepsia* **52,** 386–392.

Riva, D., Vago, C., Pantaleoni, C., Bulgheroni, S., Mantegazza, M. & Franceschetti, S. (2009): Progressive neurocognitive decline in two children with Dravet syndrome, *de novo SCN1A* truncations and different epileptic phenotypes. *Am. J. Med. Genet. A.* **149,** 2339-2345.

Wolff, M., Cassé-Perrot, C. & Dravet, C. (2006): Severe myoclonic epilepsy of infants (Dravet syndrome): natural history and neuropsychological findings. *Epilepsia* **47**(2), 45–48.

Chapter 4

The neuropsychological profile of childhood focal idiopathic epilepsy syndromes

Chiara Vago, Sara Bulgheroni, Silvia Esposito, Arianna Usilla and Daria Riva

Developmental Neurology Division, Fondazione IRCCS Istituto Neurologico 'C. Besta',
via Celoria 11, 20133 Milan, Italy
neuropsicologia@istituto-besta.it

Summary

Focal idiopathic epilepsy syndromes are the most common forms of childhood-related epilepsy in children between 3 and 12 years of age and include benign rolandic epilepsy, benign epilepsy with occipital paroxysms (Gastaut syndrome), and Panayiotopoulos syndrome. These syndromes are characterized by epileptic activity originating in a specific brain area, a high degree of familial clustering, age-related progression, psychomotor development at onset within the normal range, negative neuroimaging findings, a generally good response to pharmacological therapy, and spontaneous remission at adolescence.

Based on studies of children with the rolandic form, as well as on the fewer numbers of paediatric patients with occipital paroxysms, mild neuropsychological deficits with dysfunction in different areas of functioning have been described. Deficits in language skills, academic learning, mnestic abilities, and visual motor and attention-executive skills have generally been described. In particular, in connection with the site of electroencephalographic abnormalities, and as far as the rolandic form is concerned, a large number of findings provide support for an impairment in language and mnestic skills prevalently with regard to verbal material and various degrees and forms of learning disabilities. With regards to early and late-onset occipital epilepsies, deficits primarily of visual-perception function and attention skills have been described.

Introduction

Focal idiopathic epilepsy syndromes are the most common forms of childhood-related epilepsy in children between 3 and 12 years of age (Panayiotopoulos *et al.*, 2008). Idiopathic focal epilepsies can be divided in two groups: non-autosomal dominant and autosomal dominant (Vigevano *et al.*, 2013). Non-autosomal dominant entities include benign epilepsy with centrotemporal spikes or rolandic epilepsy (BECTS), idiopathic childhood occipital epilepsy of Gastaut (ICOE-G), and Panayiotopoulos syndrome (PS). When PS was recently formally recognized as a nosographic entity of its own, the previously used descriptive term 'early-onset occipital epilepsy' was abandoned in favour of the new nomenclature (Berg *et al.*, 2010).

BECTS, ICOE-G, and PS share some common characteristics, such as: (1) onset during developmental age; (2) the absence of any neurological or psychomotor/cognitive developmental deficits before the onset of epileptic abnormalities; (3) familial clustering of epilepsy in a third of patients; (4) sporadic focal seizures; (5) age-related disease progression and benign evolution with remission during adolescence; and (6) specific abnormal electroencephalographic (EEG) recordings (Vigevano et al., 2013).

In view of their common characteristics, some have proposed that these epileptic symptoms be grouped under the wider heading of 'benign childhood seizure susceptibility syndrome', for patients with an idiopathic predisposition to focal seizures and/or EEG abnormalities (Panayiotopoulos et al., 2008; Vigevano et al., 2013).

Partial epilepsy with centrotemporal spikes or rolandic epilepsy (BECTS)

BECTS is better known as the most common childhood-related form of focal idiopathic epilepsy and accounts for approximately 15 per cent of all childhood forms of epilepsy (Shields & Snead, 2009). EEG tracings typically show focal centrotemporal abnormalities that can secondarily generalize with normal background activity. Seizures are few and take place during the night. Onset is usually between 3 and 10 years of age, with a peak between 5 and 8 (Dalla Bernardina et al., 2005). Prognosis is good and characterized by EEG normalization and spontaneous remission by puberty (Panayiotopoulos et al., 2008). For the greater part, BECTS patients do not require pharmacological treatment; however, if prescribed, the response is generally good (Guerrini & Pellacani, 2012). The pathogenesis of the disease is probably linked to genetic factors; the first positive evidence for linkage in families with centrotemporal spikes was found on chromosome 15q14 (Neubauer, 1998), however, studies have since not confirmed this finding (Vadlamudi et al., 2006).

BECTS: neuropsychological profile

Numerous studies have investigated neuropsychological deficits in children in an active phase of BECTS. Functional areas linked to mnestic, executive attention, visual perception abilities, and, in particular, linguistic skills and academic learning have been evaluated. It is not, however, always possible to compare the results because the tests used were not always the same; not all studies had control groups or used national norms, and only some made a covariate for IQ to assess if it is a specific deficit. With regards to global cognitive capacities, in the majority of cases, the quotients reported were found to be within the average range (Deonna, 2000; Northcott et al., 2005), although the scores tended to be lower than those of control subjects (Weglage et al., 1997; Baglietto et al., 2001; Northcott et al., 2007; Riva et al., 2007; Goldberg-Stern et al., 2010).

As already explained, linguistic abilities represent the most frequently studied functional domain also with regards to the proximity to the epileptic focus typical of BECTS, involving areas in charge of verbal input processing. A large number of studies have produced a growing body of evidence demonstrating language impairments, but the syndrome's functional profile is not yet entirely clear. In general, what has primarily been described are specific impairments in tests implicating verbal production and deficits both in basic linguistic abilities (syntax, semantics, and phonology) (Staden et al., 1998; Monjauze et al., 2005; Northcott et al., 2005; Riva et al., 2007; Verrotti et al., 2011), as well as in higher order linguistic skills (the use of language to formulate and organize one's thoughts for a coherent presentation) (Staden et al., 1998;

Lillywhite *et al.*, 2009). When our group analyzed the intellectual ability and linguistic skills of 24 children with BECTS and 16 age-matched controls (Riva *et al.*, 2007), we found that the former showed preserved naming skills but lower scores on phonemic fluency, verbal re-elaboration of semantic knowledge, and lexical comprehension. Using Clinical evaluation of Language Fundamentals, Dutch edition (Semel *et al.*, 2010), Overvliet and colleagues (2013a) found that children with BECTS had more serious impairments in semantic language processing with respect to the controls in both receptive and productive language skills.

Another interesting line of research concerns the effects of rolandic spikes on functional language lateralization. As early as 1988, Piccirilli and collaborators investigated language organization in 22 right-handed BECTS children, 14 of whom had a left-sided and 8 a right-sided electroencephalographic focus (Piccirilli *et al.*, 1988). On the basis of study findings, the authors concluded that epileptiform activity in BECTS can modify language lateralization and hypothesized that there is a bihemispheric representation. Hommet and colleagues (2001) outlined similar results in 23 adolescents and young adults in complete remission from BECTS and hypothesized that there is a long-term, persistent hemispheric language representation disorder in that population. Based on a study of 24 children with BECTS and 16 age-, gender-, and school-matched controls, our research group found an atypical performance on dichotic listening tests in the former with loss of the right ear/left hemisphere advantage, associated with a functional right ear/left hemisphere advantage characteristic of age-matched controls. Although our finding does not reflect a complete rightward shift but the loss of the advantage of one hemisphere over the other, it suggests that left hemispheric processing superiority regarding phonological stimuli is functionally disturbed by interictal spikes in these patients, leading to a bihemispheric representation of the phonological processing of verbal and nonverbal stimuli (Bulgheroni *et al.*, 2008).

Learning difficulties, which are frequently noted in children with BECTS, are likewise evaluated in relation to the patient's neuropsychological impairment in general and, in particular, to their linguistic impairment. There is substantial agreement that these children have impairment in writing, reading (Staden *et al.*, 1998; Papavasiliou *et al.*, 2005; Piccinelli *et al.*, 2008; Fonseca *et al.*, 2009), spelling (Staden *et al.*, 1998; Monjauze *et al.*, 2005; Papavasiliou *et al.*, 2005; Northcott *et al.*, 2005, 2007), and mathematics (Miziara *et al.*, 2012), although the studies considering these last two domains are less numerous. It is to be noted, nevertheless, that the type of testing and scoring methods used are not always specified which makes it difficult to compare the results of different studies and to verify how those capacities were impaired. Few studies specify which variables the deficit concerns (for example speed and/or accuracy in reading) (Monjauze *et al.*, 2005; Chaix *et al.*, 2006; Ay *et al.*, 2009) and/or the type(s) of stimuli utilized (lists of words, reading passages, calculations, or mathematical problems) (Monjauze *et al.*, 2005; Ebus *et al.*, 2011; Miziara *et al.*, 2012; Overvliet *et al.*, 2011; Smith *et al.*, 2012).

Memory also appears to be negatively influenced by spikes in the centrotemporal area (for a review, see Verrotti *et al.*, 2014); there have been reports of impairment in both verbal short-term (Weglage *et al.*, 1997; Danielsson & Petermann, 2009; Northcott *et al.*, 2005) and visuo-spatial memory (Baglietto *et al.*, 2001; Volkl-Kernstock *et al.*, 2006; Danielsson & Petermann, 2009), and also in long-term verbal memory (Northcott *et al.*, 2005), as well as in learning verbal information (Croona *et al.*, 1999; Staden *et al.*, 1998). We investigated verbal learning and retrieval and learning strategy usage using the California Verbal learning Test-Children's Version (CVLT-C). While the patients younger than 10 showed significantly worse supraspan skills and were less efficient in using a semantic clustering strategy to improve their learning than their age-matched controls, there was no difference between the over 10-year-olds and their matched controls. This finding suggests that the capacity for spontaneously using more efficient strategies matures later in BECTS children (Vago *et al.*, 2008).

Studies on executive functions identified mild deficits in information processing (D'Alessandro *et al.*, 1990; Baglietto *et al.*, 2001), inhibitory processes (Deltour *et al.*, 2007a., 2008), problem solving (Croona *et al.*, 1999), cognitive flexibility (Croona *et al.*, 1999; Deltour *et al.*, 2007b; Gunduz *et al.*, 1999), and auditory attention (Ay *et al.*, 2009) in children with BECTS.

With regards to attention skills, a review by Kavros and colleagues (2008) focusing on studies utilizing the Posner paradigm outlined deficits in attentional shifts, orientation, and executive control in these children. It is important to remember that few of the studies included in the review utilized tests that investigated all of the functions of the attention system, moreover, the samples appeared heterogenous and there was not always a clear distinction between children with attention difficulties and those diagnosed with attention deficit hyperactivity disorder (ADHD) according to the criteria of the Diagnostic and Statistical Manual of Mental Disorders Fifth edition (DSM-V; American Psychiatric Association, 2013), resulting in a heterogenous neuropsychological profile as far as the attention domain was concerned.

Cerminara and collaborators (2010) utilized a computerized test battery to evaluate attention ability in children with BECTS and found, with respect to control subjects, an impairment in different aspects of selective attention (impulsivity, focused attention, selective attention, and divided attention) and in the measure of intensity of attention (arousal), but not in the vigilance level.

Higher levels of distractibility, impulsivity, and hyperactivity have often been reported (Metz-Lutz *et al.*, 1999; Massa *et al.*, 2001; Giordani *et al.*, 2006) in studies investigating the behaviour of children with BECTS; these findings confirm neuropsychological data outlining a deficit in attention-executive ability with impairment in response inhibition and the ability to inhibit irrelevant responses.

Children with typical BECTS and a matched control group were evaluated by Volkl-Kernstock and collaborators (Volkl-Kernstock *et al.*, 2009) using the Child Behaviour Checklist (Achenbach, 1991). The patients were found to be anxious, to possess low self-esteem levels, to have difficulty in socializing with classmates and controlling disattention, and impulsive/aggressive behaviours. Using the same instrument, Holtmann and colleagues (2006) found that the presence of the centrotemporal epileptic abnormality was associated with worse symptoms in children with ADHD, favouring more impulsive behaviour, often linked to an inability or difficulty associated with inhibition (Nigg, 2000).

The problems transversally described by the studies cited, such as difficulty in verbal fluency tasks and in the strategic organization of verbal incoming material and behavioural features, such as impulsivity and lack of inhibition, confirm impairment in tasks of an executive order and point in the direction of frontal lobe dysfunction. It can be hypothesized then that, despite the typical epileptic focus in BECTS, prevalently concentrated in the central regions, variations in its propagation can interfere with the activities of other cortical regions, such as the frontal lobe, resulting in a dysfunction, apparently not strictly correlated to the site of the syndrome's epileptic focus.

Neuroimaging studies are the link between the neural architecture underlying linguistic processing and the impairment founded by neuropsychological tests. Structural magnetic resonance imaging (MRI) has detected reduced cortical thickness in left perisylvian regions in 24 children with BECTS between 8 and 14 years of age (Overvliet *et al.*, 2013b). Functional magnetic resonance imaging (fMRI) studies have revealed that language-related activation is less lateralized in BECTS subjects and that there is a reorganization of the most bilateral networks or of the right side, particularly in the anterior brain areas (Lillywhite *et al.*, 2009; Datta *et al.*, 2013; Vannest *et al.*, 2013). Volumetric brain studies have identified anomalies in frontal lobe growth; similar to controls, the prefrontal-to-frontal lobe volume ratio was reported to increase serially in BECTS subjects with normal cognitive/behavioural functioning, while it was stagnant or decreased in BECTS patients with neuropsychological problems (Kanemura *et al.*, 2011). Besseling and collaborators (2013) found a reduced functional connectivity between the sensorimotor network and the left inferior frontal gyrus in children with BECTS. These data provide further confirmation that epileptic activity in the centrotemporal area interferes with the development of dominance of the left hemisphere in processing stimuli of a linguistic nature and underline the importance of the interaction of Broca's area with the surrounding brain areas, such as the frontal area for tasks which requires planning, for example, producing phrases and denominations.

Ever greater attention is being dedicated to efforts to determine which EEG characteristics and clinical variables can be considered markers of cognitive and neuropsychological impairment. It can be inferred from studies in the literature that there is substantial agreement among investigators in favour of a negative correlation between the early onset of epileptic abnormalities and neuropsychological outcome. Seizure onset before the age of eight and epileptiform discharges (in more than 50 per cent of sleep EEG recordings) in several tracings over the period of a year are important markers which identify patients at risk of developing academic difficulties (Piccinelli *et al.*, 2008). Deltour *et al.* (2007b) found that children with an earlier onset of seizures made more omission errors and had slower reaction times in the Continuous Performance Test (CPT), and Jurkeviciene and colleagues (2012) confirmed this correlation also with reference to the linguistic domain.

Although some studies found that the nature of the impairments detected by neuropsychological testing in BECTS patients correlated with the side of the epileptic focus (Piccirilli *et al.*, 1994; Massa *et al.*, 2001; Wolff *et al.*, 2005), others found no such relationship (Deltour *et al.*, 2007b; Vago *et al.*, 2008). Studies investigating language functions using standard tests also failed to confirm any major impairment in children with a left-sided focus (Weglage *et al.*, 1997; Staden *et al.*, 1998; Metz-Lutz *et al.*, 1999; Northcott *et al.*, 2005; Jurkeviciene *et al.*, 2012). Conversely, Riva and collaborators (2007) found that children with a left-sided focus scored significantly worse than controls on phonemic fluency, while children with a right-sided focus scored significantly worse than controls in the vocabulary subtest of the Weschsler Intelligence Scale for Children, revised edition (WISC-R), and in a lexical comprehension test.

Correlating the topography of the focus (in terms of its side and localization) with neuropsychological impairments is particularly difficult in BECTS patients because spike location varies as the disorder evolves (Pinton *et al.*, 2006); there have also been reports of bilateral oscillations for lateralized time-domain spikes, suggesting a synchronized activity in a network of bilateral rolandic neurons (Lin *et al.*, 2006). Variations in spike locations in one or both hemispheres may, in fact, mean that BECTS results from a widespread age-related hyper-excitability of the sensorimotor and latero-temporal cortices, the prominent location of which varies over time leading to a functional modification that gives rise to a mild but protracted dysfunction of fine cortical processing (Kellaway, 2000). According to Metz-Lutz and colleagues (1999), epilepsy appears to disrupt response organization rather than lateralized cognitive functions, and to interfere with the development of cortical areas distant from the rolandic focus.

Multifocal anomalies appear to interfere with both linguistic (Riva *et al.*, 2007) and cognitive (Wolff *et al.*, 2005) performance and have a particularly significant impact on the laterality index with a complete loss of the right-ear advantage, in favour of symmetric performance (Bulgheroni *et al.*, 2008). These results may mean that widespread hyperexcitability is capable of causing more severe disruption.

Published data are discordant with regards to the correlation between spike frequency and neuropsychological function. IQ deficits were, nevertheless, found to be significantly correlated with the frequency of EEG spikes (Weglage *et al.*, 1997; Riva *et al.*, 2007). Staden and collaborators (1998) reported that there is a tendency towards worse language dysfunction when epileptic discharges are more frequent. Conversely, Massa and colleagues (2001) found no direct cause-and-effect relationship between the number of interictal paroxysms and cognitive symptoms, although the mean number of such paroxysms differed in statistical terms in the typical and complicated groups studied. Northcott and collaborators (2005) found no correlation between spike burden and memory difficulties or phonological awareness. Weglage and colleagues (1997) quantified spike frequency but they did not find it to be correlated with specific neuropsychological or language functions. Bulgheroni and colleagues (2008), instead, found no significant correlation between dichotic listening performance and the interictal discharge rate, and hypothesized that cortical dysfunctional states depend on protracted periods of hyperexcitability leading to centrotemporal spikes, rather than on the time course (and quantity) of the spikes at the time of assessment. It could be argued that the lack of any correlation between the spike rate and neuropsychological data could be due to the fact that the EEG recording used to calculate the interictal spike rate and the neuropsychological assessment were too far apart in time to allow for accurate analysis. However, Wolff *et al.* (2005), who conducted a combined EEG/magentoencephalography (MEG) examination at around the same time as a neuropsychological assessment, found no correlation between the spike rate and cognitive performance.

Many authors of longitudinal studies have described an improvement in neuropsychological function comparable to levels found in control subjects at the time corresponding to remission of epileptiform activity (D'Alessandro *et al.*, 1990; Metz-Lutz *et al.*, 1999; Deonna *et al.*, 2000; Baglietto *et al.*, 2001; Hommet *et al.*, 2001; Lindgren *et al.*, 2004; Northcott *et al.*, 2006; Volkl-Kernstock *et al.*, 2009; Callenbach *et al.*, 2010). Recently, evidence demonstrating that neuropsychological impairment continues after EEG recordings have normalized has been reported. Although in a limited number of subjects, Monjauze and collaborators (2011) found a specific impairment in receptive vocabulary, sentence assembly, expressive language, and basic reading abilities that persisted after the active phase of the seizure disorder. They concluded that epileptic activity in the centrotemporal region during developmental age can have a permanent effect on brain and language development. Filippini and colleagues (2013) studied 18 children with BECTS aged between 8 and 18. During the study's follow-up period, they found an impairment in linguistic and mnestic abilities, characterized by an inferior digit span, difficulty in phonological coding in lexical access, and attention problems, that persisted to the time of the final evaluation. However, only a few studies have examined neuropsychological function after epileptic abnormalities have ceased and only a few subjects have been evaluated. The temporal interval between the evaluation and normalization of EEG recordings has, moreover, been variable and thus not comparable. Further confirmation is thus necessary before it can be ascertained whether BECTS constitutes the aetiological basis of neuropyschological difficulties or whether interictal epileptic activity affects cognitive development and, in particular, the consolidation of verbal skills.

Panayiotopoulos syndrome

Panayiotopoulos syndrome (PS) is a common, childhood-related, autonomic epilepsy. Its EEG pattern is characterized by a marked variability in the localization of spikes; the abnormalities are normally multifocal and frequently localized to the occipital lobe. Age at onset is frequently between 1 and 14 years of age, with a peak between 4 and 5 years; seizures are generally infrequent but long-lasting with autonomic manifestations (Vigevano *et al.*, 2013). The prevalence of PS is still uncertain as the syndrome has only recently been formally recognized; the clinical manifestations are similar to typical manifestations of other pathological conditions and the syndrome is often characterized by a single episode (Panayiotopoulos *et al.*, 2008; Michael *et al.*, 2010). Prognosis is good. As far as a genetic aetiology is concerned, a mutation of the *SCN1A* gene (Livingston *et al.*, 2009) has been reported, but not confirmed by successive studies (Panayiotopoulos, 2010).

Idiopathic childhood occipital epilepsy of Gastaut

Idiopathic childhood occipital epilepsy of Gastaut (ICOE-G) is a form of idiopathic occipital epilepsy accounting for approximately 2 to 7 per cent of the idiopathic childhood epilepsies (Taylor *et al.*, 2008). The interictal EEG shows characteristic occipital paroxysms (Ferrari-Marinho *et al.*, 2013). Onset is typically later than that of PS which characteristically occurs between 3 and 16 years of age, with a peak between 8 and 11. Seizures are generally diurnal and frequent, although short lasting, and symptoms are visual including, in particular, visual hallucinations and/or blindness (Adcock & Panayiotopoulos, 2012). Studies indicate that 21 per cent to 37 per cent of patients with ICOE-G have a family history of epilepsy and 9 per cent to 16 per cent of migraine headaches, but familial ICOE-G is rare (Panayiotopoulos *et al.*, 2008; Caraballo *et al.*, 2009). Prognosis is uncertain and the data available indicate that remission takes place in 50-60 per cent of patients within 2-4 years of disease onset (Caraballo *et al.*, 2007). ICOE-G often requires pharmacological treatment because, although brief and mild, the seizures are frequent, and a secondary generalized form may be inevitable without treatment (Panayiotopoulos *et al.*, 2008; Vigevano *et al.*, 2013).

ICOE-G and PS: neuropsychological profile

Fewer neuropsychological studies have been carried out in children with PS or ICOE-G with respect to investigations in patients with BECTS. Over time, a more precise profile defining more homogeneous samples from a diagnostic viewpoint has been formed by virtue of the recent recognition of PS as a diagnostic entity of its own. While producing the first important results in this line of research, the studies cited here require further confirmatory data in view of the low number of samples studied, the non-comparability between studies with regards to the diagnostic criteria utilized to subdivide the samples, and the presence of studies considering only the active phase of the disorder.

With regards to cognitive capacities, even children with prevalently occipital forms appear, for the most part, to have abilities within the normal range, although they tend to be lower with respect to control subjects (Gulgonen *et al.*, 2000; Germanò *et al.*, 2005; Chilosi *et al.*, 2006). In the majority of cases, non-verbal performance scores are inferior with respect to verbal performance scores (Gulgonen *et al.*, 2000; Germanò *et al.*, 2005; Gagliano *et al.*, 2007; Polat *et al.*, 2012), and there are more frequent deficits in the Picture Completion, Imagined Stories, and Object Reconstruction subtests of the Wechsler Scale. A smaller number of studies have not, however, confirmed this functional pattern (Chilosi *et al.*, 2006; Specchio *et al.*, 2010).

With regards to neuropsychological functioning, there is substantial evidence that there is a great deal of vulnerability associated with high-level visual processing; children with occipital epilepsy have, in fact, deficits in facial discrimination (Chilosi *et al.*, 2006), impaired visual object identification (Brancati *et al.*, 2012), and altered coherence thresholds of form perception (De Rose *et al.*, 2010). Results concerning verbal, academic, memory, and visual motor integration abilities are, instead, discordant. Polat and colleagues (2012), who subdivided a sample relative to the time at onset of epileptic abnormalities (late or early), found that children with late onset had impairments in visual spatial perception and visual motor integration, but not in verbal and visual short-term memory. By assessing voluntary orientation and reorientation of visual spatial attention in patients with BECTS and PS, and healthy controls, Bedoin and collaborators (2012) found different attentional deficiencies depending on the form of the epileptic syndrome; children with right-sided BECTS showed a strong tendency towards a rightward bias in attentional orientation, children with comorbid ADHD showed unilateral deficits of disengagement, and children with PS failed to diffuse inhibition except in the nearest area outside the attentional focus. Hirano and colleagues (2009) designed a restrospective study investigating a larger sample relative to other studies (79 children with PS) and subdivided subjects depending on the number of seizures they had experienced: typical PS (seizure recurrence: 1-5 times), borderline (6-9 times), and atypical PS (> 10 times). The authors found no significant difference between the three groups with regards to cognitive capacity, but noted a greater frequency of neurodevelopmental and behavioural disorders in the group with the largest number of seizures.

Conclusions

Paediatric epileptic disorders can interfere with normal neurocognitive development; the precise nature and severity of neuropsychological deficits vary depending on the specific localization, diffusion, and severity of epileptic discharges.

Summarizing the findings emerging from the studies examined, we can conclude that children with focal idiopathic epilepsy syndromes tend to show a lower global intelligence quotient although within normal parameters. We can thus hypothesize that these syndromes cause a general reduction in the cognitive potential of these patients. Generally speaking, centrotemporal epilepsy disorders predominantly compromise neuropsychological functions belonging to the verbal domain with greater impairment in verbal and phonological production and academic learning. Occipital area epilepsies, instead, appear to predominantly compromise visual perception and attention. A wide range of deficits have in any case been described and a co-occurrence of different types of neuropsychological deficits is clearly evident; further studies are necessary to shed light on the cause-effect relationships between deficits in the different neuropsychological domains (Verrotti *et al.*, 2014).

Impairments in neuropsychological abilities not processed classically by the areas in which the epileptic spike foci are predominant have been described; it would appear then that despite the fact that the epileptic foci are prevalently concentrated in centrotemporal and occipital regions, variations in their propagation can interfere with the activities of adjacent brain areas, causing wider neuropsychological deficits.

Impairment is correlated to age at onset and to the severity of EEG abnormalities; early presenting spikes and diffuse epileptic disorders interfere in a significant way with brain maturation and in the development of capacities processed by the affected areas, and determine worse neuropsychological performance.

The neuropsychological impairment described here, which does not appear to compromise daily function, is in any case considered mild, and a thorough neuropsychological evaluation is necessary to identify the deficits involved and investigate the individual functional profile of these children.

Conflicts of interest: none.

References

Achenbach, T.M. *Manual for the Child Behavior Checklist/4-8 and 1991 profile (1991)*. Burlington, VT: University of Vermont, Department of Psychiatry, University of Vermont; 1991.

Adcock, J.E. & Panayiotopoulos, C.P. (2012): Occipital lobe seizures and epilepsies. *J. Clin. Neurophysiol.* **29**, 397–407.

American Psychiatric Association. (2013). *Diagnostic and Statistical Manual of Mental Disorders, Fifth Edition.* Arlington, VA, American Psychiatric Association, Web. (Access date: 1 June 2013). dsm.psychiatryonline.org.

Ay, Y., Gokben, S., Serdaroglu, G., et al. (2009): Neuropsychologic impairment in children with rolandic epilepsy. *Pediatr. Neurol.* **41**, 359–363.

Baglietto, M.G., Battaglia, F.M., Nobili, L., et al. (2001): Neuropsychological disorders related to interictal epileptic discharges during sleep in benign epilepsy of childhood with centrotemporal or Rolandic spikes. *Dev. Med. Child Neurol.* **43**, 407–412.

Bedoin, N., Ciumas, C., Lopez, C., et al. (2012): Disengagement and inhibition of visual-spatial attention are differently impaired in children with rolandic epilepsy and Panayiotopoulos syndrome. *Epilepsy Behav.* **25**, 81–91.

Berg, A.T., Berkovic, S.F., Brodie, M.J., et al. (2010): Revised terminology and concepts for organization of seizures and epilepsies: report of the ILAE Commission on Classification and Terminology, 2005-2009. *Epilepsia* **51**, 676–685.

Besseling, R.M., Jansen, J.F., Overvliet, G.M., et al. (2013): Reduced functional integration of the sensorimotor and language network in rolandic epilepsy. *Neuroimage Clin.* **2**, 239–246.

Brancati, C., Barba, C., Metitieri, T., et al. (2012): Impaired object identification in idiopathic childhood occipital epilepsy. *Epilepsia* **53**, 686–694.

Bulgheroni, S., Franceschetti, S., Vago, C., et al. (2008): Verbal dichotic listening performance and its relationship with EEG features in benign childhood epilepsy with centrotemporal spikes. *Epilepsy Res.* **79**, 31–38.

Callenbach, P.M., Bouma, P.A., Geerts, A.T., et al. (2010): Long-term outcome of benign childhood epilepsy with centrotemporal spikes: Dutch Study of Epilepsy in Childhood. *Seizure* **19**, 501–506.

Caraballo, R., Cerosino, R. & Fejerman, N. (2007): Panayiotopoulos syndrome: a prospective study of 192 patients. *Epilepsia* **48**, 1054–1061.

Caraballo, R., Koutroumanidis, M., Panayiotopoulos, C.P. & Fejerman, N. (2009): Idiopathic childhood occipital epilepsy of Gastaut: a review and differentiation from migraine and other epilepsies. *J. Child Neurol.* **24**, 1536–1542.

Cerminara, C., D'Agati, E., Lange, K.W., et al. (2010): Benign childhood epilepsy with centrotemporal spikes and the multicomponent model of attention: a matched control study. *Epilepsy Behav.* **19**, 69–77.

Chaix, Y., Laguitton, V., Lauwers-Cances, V., et al. (2006): Reading abilities and cognitive functions of children with epilepsy: influence of epileptic syndrome. *Brain Dev.* **28**, 122–130.

Chilosi, A.M., Brovedani, P., Moscatelli, M., Bonanni, P. & Guerrini, R. (2006): Neuropsychological findings in idiopathic occipital lobe epilepsies. *Epilepsia* **47**(2), 76–78.

Croona, C., Kihlgren, M., Lundberg, S., Eeg-Olofsson, O. & Eeg-Olofsson, K.E. (1999): Neuropsychological findings in children with benign childhood epilepsy with centrotemporal spikes. *Dev. Med. Child Neurol.* **41**, 813–818.

D'Alessandro, P., Piccirilli, M., Tiacci, C., et al. (1990): Neuropsychological features of benign partial epilepsy in children. *Ital. J. Neurol. Sci.* **11**, 265–269.

Riva, D., Vago, C., Franceschetti, S., et al. (2007): Intellectual and language findings and their relationship to EEG characteristics in benign childhood epilepsy with centrotemporal spikes. *Epilepsy Behav.* **10,** 278–285.

Shields, W.D. & Snead, O.C.3rd (2009): Benign epilepsy with centrotemporal spikes. *Epilepsia* **50**(8), 10–15.

Smith, A.B., Kavros, P.M., Clarke, T., Dorta, N.J., Tremont, G. & Pal, D.K. (2012): A neurocognitive endophenotype associated with rolandic epilepsy. *Epilepsia* **53,** 705–711.

Specchio, N., Trivisano, M., Di Ciommo, V., et al. (2010): Panayiotopoulos syndrome: a clinical, EEG, and neuropsychological study of 93 consecutive patients. *Epilepsia* **51,** 2098–2107.

Staden, U., Isaacs, E., Boyd, S.G., Brandl, U. & Neville, B.G. (1998): Language dysfunction in children with Rolandic epilepsy. *Neuropediatrics* **29,** 242–248.

Taylor, I., Berkovic, S.F., Kivity, S. & Scheffer, I.E. (2008): Benign occipital epilepsies of childhood: clinical features and genetics. *Brain* **131,** 2287–2294.

Vadlamudi, L., Kjeldsen, M.J., Corey, L.A., et al. (2006): Analyzing the etiology of benign rolandic epilepsy: a multicenter twin collaboration. *Epilepsia* **47,** 550–555.

Vago, C., Bulgheroni, S., Franceschetti, S., Usilla, A. & Riva, D. (2008): Memory performance on the California Verbal Learning Test of children with benign childhood epilepsy with centrotemporal spikes. *Epilepsy Behav.* **13,** 600–606.

Vannest, J., Szaflarski, J.P., Eaton, K.P., et al. (2013): Functional magnetic resonance imaging reveals changes in language localization in children with benign childhood epilepsy with centrotemporal spikes. *J. Child Neurol.* **28,** 435–445.

Verrotti, A., D'Egidio, C., Agostinelli, S., Parisi, P., Chiarelli, F. & Coppola, G. (2011): Cognitive and linguistic abnormalities in benign childhood epilepsy with centrotemporal spikes. *Acta Paediatr.* **100,** 768–772.

Verrotti, A., Filippini, M., Matricardi, S., Agostinelli, M.F. & Gobbi, G. (2014): Memory impairment and benign epilepsy with centrotemporal spikes (BECTS): a growing suspicion. *Brain Cogn.* **84,** 123–131.

Vigevano, F., Specchio, N. & Fejerman, N. (2013): Idiopathic focal epilepsies. *Handb. Clin. Neurol.* **111,** 591–604.

Volkl-Kernstock, S., Willinger, U. & Feucht, M. (2006): Spacial perception and spatial memory in children with benign childhood epilepsy with centro-temporal spikes (BCECTS). *Epilepsy Res.* **72,** 39–48.

Volkl-Kernstock, S., Bauch-Prater, S., Ponocny-Seliger, E. & Feucht, M. (2009): Speech and school performance in children with benign partial epilepsy with centro-temporal spikes (BCECTS). *Seizure* **18,** 320–326.

Weglage, J., Demsky, A., Pietsch, M. & Kurlemann, G. (1997): Neuropsychological, intellectual, and behavioral findings in patients with centrotemporal spikes with and without seizures. *Dev. Med. Child Neurol.* **39,** 646–651.

Wolff, M., Weiskopf, N., Serra, E., Preissl, H., Birbaumer, N. & Kraegeloh-Mann, I. (2005): Benign partial epilepsy in childhood: selective cognitive deficits are related to the location of focal spikes determined by combined EEG/MEG. *Epilepsia* **46,** 1661–1667.

Chapter 5

Lesional epilepsies in childhood: neuropsychological and psychopathological aspects

Valentina Sibilia and Renzo Guerrini

Paediatric Neurology Unit and Laboratories, Children's Hospital A. Meyer, University of Florence,
viale Pieraccini 24, 50139 Florence, Italy
r.guerrini@meyer.it

Summary

The potential for a curative effect of epilepsy surgery in children with medically intractable epilepsy has led to ever expanding research on postoperative cognitive and behavioural outcome. However, the multiple dependent variables which may influence neuropsychological outcome in epilepsy surgery are difficult to uncouple. Factors such as age at seizure onset, aetiology, age at surgery, concomitant drug treatment, type of surgical approach, and seizure frequency may need to be considered when examining the outcome and should be analyzed in a multivariate manner. Furthermore, paediatric neuropsychological research, examining the impact of epilepsy surgery, has focused on intellectual functioning with only a few investigations addressing specific neuropsychological functions in a long-term perspective. In spite of a limited number of impressive observations of recovery of cognitive abilities after surgical treatment, overall, no conclusive evidence on cognitive outcome has been obtained and only a few elements emerge from the available studies, all limited by the small sample size and lack of adequate control groups.

Introduction

It has been suggested that chronic epilepsy generally impairs cognition and also induces processes of functional reorganization and behavioural compensations (Elger *et al.*, 2004). Poor cognitive outcome is generally associated with early onset, long duration, and poor seizure control (Helmstaedter *et al.*, 2001). In selected candidates, surgery for epilepsy can be beneficial, ameliorating or significantly decreasing seizures from 50 to 80 per cent, according to aetiology and areas involved (Obeid *et al.*, 2009). In order to investigate the cognitive consequences of epilepsy surgery in children, neuropsychological assessment is an essential part of the pre and post-operative work-up.

Neuropsychological and behavioural aspects

The extent of a brain lesion is a conditioning factor in cognitive development; children with large lesions in multiple lobes are more likely to manifest global deficits than those whose lesions extend only to the frontal or temporal lobe (Freitag & Tuxhorn, 2005). Vasconcellos and collaborators (2001) suggested that early seizure onset is linked to a significantly higher occurrence of intellectual disability, regardless of the subtype of lesion. In contrast, Westerveld and colleagues (2000) and Skirrow and collaborators (2011) could not identify age at seizure onset as a predictor of cognitive functioning.

Frontal lobe epilepsy

Frontal lobe epilepsy (FLE) has the potential to impact a wide range of cognitive domains. Children with FLE show impairments in executive functions, (Riva et al., 2005; Hernandez et al., 2003; Culhane-Shelburne et al., 2002), motor coordination (Lendt et al., 2002), and attention deficit, often associated with difficulties in computing skills. Cohen and Le Normand (1998) noted a clear dissociation in linguistic performances between comprehension and production in children with left frontal epileptogenic foci who exhibited early deficiencies in language comprehension. Linguistic comprehension was initially impaired but gradually improved to reach normal performance levels by age seven. Memory deficits have, for a long time, been mainly attributed to temporal lobe epilepsy, however, one study showed that lengthy duration of active epilepsy was the leading factor for memory impairment (Nolan et al., 2004).

Several case series mention behavioural disturbances in children with FLE (Boone et al., 1988; Jambaqué & Dulac, 1989; Lassonde et al., 2000; Lagae et al., 2001; Riva et al., 2002; Auclair et al., 2005; Prévost et al., 2006; Derry et al., 2008); the association with ADHD being the most common. Seizure frequency and poor seizure control have been proposed as risk factors associated with attention difficulties and inability to inhibit impulse responses (Jambaqué & Dulac, 1989; Lendt et al., 2002; Riva et al., 2002; Derry et al., 2008). The efficacy of seizure control in these cases suggests that a functional disturbance of brain regions involved in the regulation of attention and behaviour is responsible for these symptoms. There is a need for studies on the aetiology of FLE-associated behavioural disturbances. Various hypotheses exist. First, from a functional anatomical perspective, for example, the apparent high prevalence of behavioural disorders in children with FLE is explained by the intimate connection of frontal and temporal limbic structures (Blumer et al., 1998). Second, cognitive and behavioural problems can be the result of the epilepsy-related factors. These include the onset age of seizures, frequency of seizures, occurrence of secondary generalized attacks, and the location and extent of the epileptogenic area (Fohlen et al., 2004). Third, the association between psychosis or ictal fear and FLE has been linked to the reciprocal connections between the amygdala, the orbito-frontal and the anterior cingulated regions, as well as between the frontal and temporal lobes through the uncinate fasciculus and the superior longitudinal fasciculus (Mega et al., 1997). Fourth, aggressive behaviour has been related to activation of limbic structures and loss of frontal suppression of limbic activity and, possibly as a consequence of discharges spreading to other frontal, temporal, or limbic structures (Sumer et al., 2007).

Temporal lobe epilepsy

Memory impairment has been extensively explored in children with temporal lesions. There appears to be a link with hemispheric specificity, as demonstrated by the association between poor performance on verbal memory and left temporal lobe epilepsy and between decline of visuo-spatial memory and right temporal lobe epilepsy (Cohen, 1992). Studies on the correlation between psychopathological disorders and types of lesions established a greater vulnerability in patients with focal lesions. It is still unclear whether this predisposition is more pronounced in patients with temporal lesions. However, in a longitudinal study of 100 children with temporal lobe epilepsy, only 15 per cent were free of psychiatric disorders (Ounsted et al., 1969).

Posterior lesional epilepsy

Occipito-parietal lesions can produce visual field impairment as well as visual processing impairment due to a defect in the visual dual stream function (Battaglia et al., 2012; Gleissner et al., 2008). At pre-surgical evaluation, these patients may show impaired visuo-motor integration and a discrepancy between VIQ and PIQ. However, Gleissner and collaborators (2008) observed functional discordant deficits on the lesion side. In left PLE (parietal lobe epilepsy), such profiles could indicate a crowding effect caused by inter-hemispheric reorganization of language functions. Yet in right PLE, the observed findings are difficult to explain, particularly in patients only exhibiting verbal memory deficits.

Cognitive and neuropsychological outcomes after epilepsy surgery

There is no conclusive evidence for cognitive outcome after epilepsy surgery; although limited elements emerge from the available studies, all data are limited by the small sample size and lack of adequate control groups (Engel et al., 2003). Additionally, the majority of these studies focused on the effects of temporal lobectomy with very young children being excluded. A prospective study (Viggedal et al., 2012) reported an increase in average IQ during a time interval ranging from 2 to 10 years after surgery. Moreover, Ramantani and colleagues (2013) reported improvement in 93 per cent of thirty subjects 2 years after surgery. In a controlled study, Skirrow and collaborators (2011) compared the cognitive performance between children who had undergone temporal lobe resection and eleven children who were comparable to the surgical group with regards to drug resistance, age at seizure onset, and duration of epilepsy, although not necessarily candidates for surgery. The surgical group showed a significant increase in IQ scores only after 6 years or more, postoperatively, as also suggested by Freitag & Tuxhorn (2005).

Determinants of cognitive outcome in paediatric epilepsy surgery

The possible determinants of cognitive outcome fall into pre-surgical, surgical, and post-surgical variables.

Pre-surgical variables

Some authors do not recognize correlations between aetiology and post-surgical cognitive abilities (Jonas et al., 2004; Loddenkemper et al., 2007; D'Argenzio et al., 2011). However, in one study on cognitive outcome after hemispherectomy (Pulsifer et al., 2004), aetiology was the most significant predictor of cognitive skills at follow-up, with Rasmussen and vascular groups scoring significantly higher than the cortical dysplasia group in general intelligence and receptive language. The same profiles were confirmed at follow-up.

The age at seizure onset appears to be strongly correlated to worse outcome after extra temporal resection (D'Argenzio et al., 2011), but unrelated to outcome in temporal lobe resections (Westerveld et al., 2000; Skirrow et al., 2011).

Shorter duration of epilepsy was associated with higher post-surgical QS after hemispherectomy (Jonas et al., 2004) and higher IQ scores after extra-temporal resection (D'Argenzio et al., 2011). Duration of epilepsy was not a predictor of IQ alterations after temporal lobectomy (Miranda & Smith, 2001), or after epilepsy surgery in Sturge-Weber syndrome (Bourgeois et al., 2007).

A link between low IQ and preoperative and postoperative cognitive decline was reported by Rausch (1991). Bjørnaes and colleagues (2004) reported a decline only in children with preoperative high performance and concluded that preoperative cognitive level is not a predictor of postoperative changes. Significant improvement was also observed in the majority of children with low preoperative QS by Freitag and Tuxhorn (2005). These authors hypothesized that a global cognitive gain may indicate a resumption of development after a period of arrest or regression due to severe epilepsy. Studying children and adolescents with different degrees of cognitive impairment (IQ < 70, 71-85, and > 85), Gleissner and collaborators (2006) suggested that cognitive level did not represent an exclusion criterion for a comprehensive pre-surgical assessment because it was not a predictor of postoperative outcome in children with epilepsy.

Surgery at an earlier age (in infants and young children) appears to be associated with a greater improvement in cognitive scores after epilepsy surgery (Loddenkemper et al., 2007; Bourgeois et al., 2007; Westerveld et al., 2000). In contrast, a study of temporal lobectomies in older children (Miranda & Smith, 2001) revealed that surgery was predictive of improvement in VIQ.

Boshuisen and colleagues (2010) tested the relationship between cognitive outcome and contralateral MRI or EEG abnormalities and found that children with contralateral MRI abnormalities more often exhibited severe intellectual disability after hemispherectomy.

Surgical variables

Hemispherectomy appears to be associated with the lowest QS (Korkman et al., 2005) and the side of surgery does not appear to be related to eventual cognitive outcomes or to changes in cognitive outcome levels (Westerveld et al., 2000), while completeness of the resection can be a significant predictor of developmental improvement after surgery (Bourgeois, 2007).

Post-surgical variables

The relationship between postoperative seizure status and cognitive outcome is not statistically significant (Boshuisen et al., 2010; Loddenkemper et al., 2007; D'Argenzio et al., 2011; Freitag & Tuxhorn, 2005; Skirrow et al., 2011). Other studies (Bourgeois et al., 2007; Miranda & Smith, 2001; Lee et al., 2010) have shown a correlation between post-surgical seizure control and improved IQ and VIQ. In a study of long-term intellectual outcome after temporal lobe surgery in childhood (Skirrow et al., 2011), the withdrawal of AEDs was an independent predictor of cognitive improvement. In patients who underwent hemispherectomy, however, the number of AEDs used at postoperative neuropsychological evaluation did not differ between children who gained ten or more IQ points and those exhibiting no postoperative improvement (Boshuisen *et al.*, 2010).

Neuropsychological outcome

Along with classic studies aimed at defining possible cognitive outcomes, there are more recent studies which have explored the evolution of specific neuropsychological functions. In these studies, sample sizes vary but do not usually feature more than twenty patients each.

Compared to adults, children would be less vulnerable to memory decline after surgery with improved attention functions one year after surgery (Gleissner *et al.*, 2005). However, a decline in VIQ and verbal memory (especially in word-pair learning) has been described in children whose surgical resection included the left temporal lobe (Meekes *et al.*, 2013).

With respect to extra-temporal resections, the few available studies show greater preoperative deficits when compared to patients with temporal lesions. It has also been suggested that verbal memory may be vulnerable after extra-temporal surgery in children (Lah, 2004), although at least two studies that included children with extra-temporal resections have found no evidence of decline (Lendt *et al.*, 2002; Mabbot & Smith, 2003).

The relationship between parietal lesions and tactile/visual agnosia, apraxia, aphasia, contralateral neglect, and disorders of body image, has been well studied in adults (Siegel, 2003). For paediatric patients with parietal lobe epilepsy, only two studies, in which small samples were investigated (Battaglia *et al.*, 2012; Gleissner *et al.*, 2008), are available, both reporting improvement in performances abilities.

Behavioural aspects

Behavioural changes that follow surgical treatment are poorly known. In a study of sixty patients undergoing temporal lobe resections (McLellan, 2005), 83 per cent had a psychiatric diagnosis established on the basis of the DSM (Diagnostic and Statistical Manual of Mental Disorders)-IV. After surgery, there was no indication of a reduced rate of psychiatric illnesses, in spite of seizure freedom. In a study of fifty-one children with refractory epilepsy, conducted with the inclusion of a control group of epilepsy children who were not surgically treated (Smith *et al.*, 2004), psychological and social difficulties, present at the first evaluation, persisted after surgery. These data do not confirm the hypothesis that seizure control has a positive influence on behavioural disorders. In contrast, Lendt and colleagues (2000) reported improvements (at a significantly higher level in seizure-free patients) in internalizing, externalizing and attention scales, that were already detectable 1 year after surgery.

Conclusion

The primary objective of epilepsy surgery is to eliminate seizures (Cross *et al.*, 2006). However, postoperative outcome should not only be expressed in terms of seizure freedom, as cognitive outcome is a factor of at least the same importance (Spencer & Huh, 2008). The study of neuropsychological outcome not only serves to enhance our knowledge in basic research but is also a basis for planning speech and neuropsychological rehabilitation post-surgery. However, there is no conclusive evidence for this since not all factors may be investigated and the multiple dependent variables which may influence cognitive outcome after surgery are difficult to uncouple. Due to small sample sizes and heterogeneity of cohorts, in most studies, only descriptive statistics are possible (Van Schooneveld & Braun, 2013). Furthermore, a lack of adequate control groups represents a weakness of most epilepsy surgery studies. Controls vary substantially between studies; many subjects were not eligible for surgery and for others, no adequate clinical description was provided (Téllez-Zenteno *et al.*, 2007). In our experience, some patients do exhibit a remarkable post-operative improvement in cognitive skills and behaviour after operation, if worthwhile seizure improvement is achieved. However, neuropsychological outcome with respect to the pre-operative status is highly unpredictable. Multicentric studies with large series of patients represent a real opportunity to resolve some of the limitations most studies have until now faced.

Conflicts of interest: none.

References

Auclair, L., Jambaqué, I., Dulac, O., La Berge, D. & Siéroff, E. (2005): Deficit of preparatory attention in children with frontal lobe epilepsy. *Neuropsychologia* **43**, 1701–1712.

Battaglia, D., Chieffo, D., Tamburrini, G., *et al.* (2012): Posterior resection for childood epilepsy: Neuropsychological evolution. *Epilepsy Behav.* **23**, 131–137.

Bjørnaes, H., Stabell, K.E., Heminghyt, E., Røste, G.K. & Bakke, S.J. (2004): Resective surgery for intractable focal epilepsy in patients with low IQ: predictors for seizure control and outcome with respect to seizures and neuropsychological and psychosocial functioning. *Epilepsia* **45**, 131–139.

Blumer, D., Wakhlu, S., Davies, K. & Hermann, B. (1998): Psychiatric outcome of temporal lobectomy for epilepsy: incidence and treatment of psychiatric complications. *Epilepsia* **39**, 478–486.

Boone, K.B., Miller, B.L., Rosenberg, L., Durazo, A., McIntyre, H. & Weil, M. (1988): Neuropsychological and behavioural abnormalities in a adolescent with frontal lobe seizure. *Neurology* **38**, 583–586.

Boshuisen, K., Van Schooneveld, M.M.J., Leijten, F.S.S., de Kort, G.A.P., van Rijen, P.C. & Gosselaar, P.H. (2010): Controlateral MRI abnormalities affect seizure and cognitive outcome after hemispherectomy. *Neurology* **75**, 1623–1630.

Bourgeois, M., Crimmins, D.W., De Oliveira, R.S., Arzimanoglou, A., Garnett, M. & Roujeau, T. (2007): Surgical treatment of epilepsy in Sturge-Weber syndrome in children. *J. Neurosurg.* **106**, 20–28.

Cohen, M. (1992): Auditory/verbal and visual/spatial memory in children with complex partial epilepsy of temporal lobe origin. *Brain Cognit.* **20**, 315–326.

Cohen, H. & Le Normand, M.T. (1998): Language development in children with simple-partial left-hemisphere epilepsy. *Brain Lang.* **64**, 583–586.

Culhane-Shelburne, K., Chapieski, L., Hiscock, M. & Glaze, D. (2002): Executive functions in children with frontal and temporal lobe epilepsy. *J. Int. Neuropsychol. Soc.* **8**, 623–632.

Cross, J.H, Jayakar, P., Nordli, D., *et al.*; International League against Epilepsy. Subcommission for Pediatric Epilepsy Surgery; Commissions of Neurosurgery and Pediatrics (2006): Proposed criteria for referral and evaluation of children for epilepsy surgery: recommendations of the Subcommission for Pediatric Epilepsy Surgery. *Epilepsia* **47**, 952–959.

D'Argenzio, L., Colonnelli, M.C., Harrison, S., Jacques, T.S., Harkness, W. & Vargha-Khadem, F. (2011): Cognitive outcome after extratemporal epilepsy surgery in childhood. *Epilepsia* **52**, 1966–1972.

Derry, C.P., Heron, S.E., Philips, F., *et al.* (2008): Severe autosomal dominant nocturnal frontal lobe epilepsy associated with psychiatric disorders and intellectual disability. *Epilepsia* **49**, 2125–2129.

Elger, C.E., Helmstaedter, C. & Kurthen, M. (2004): Chronic epilepsy and cognition. *Lancet Neurol.* **3**, 663–672.

Engel, J.J.R., Wiebe, S., French, J., *et al.*; Quality Standards Subcommittee of the American Academy of Neurology; American Epilepsy Society; American Association of Neurological Surgeons. (2003): Practice parameter: temporal lobe and localized neocortical resections for epilepsy: report of the quality Standards Subcommittee of the American Academy of Neurology, in association with the American Epilepsy Society and the American Association of Neurological Surgeons. *Neurology* **60**, 538–547.

Fohlen, M., Bulteau, C., Jalin, C., Jambaqué, I. & Delande, O. (2004): Behavioural epileptic seizures: a clinical and intracranial EEG study in 8 children with frontal lobe epilepsy. *Neuropediatrics* **35**, 336–345.

Freitag, H. & Tuxhorn, I. (2005): Cognitive function in preschool children after epilepsy surgery: rationale for early intervention. *Epilepsia* **46**, 561–567.

Gleissner, U., Clussman, H. & Sassen, R. (2006): Postsurgical outcome in pediatric patients with epilepsy: a comparison of patients with intellectual disabilities, subaverage intelligence, and average-range intelligence. *Epilepsia* **47**, 406–414.

Gleissner, U., Kuczaty, S., Clussman, H., Egler, C.E. & Helmstaedter, C. (2008): Neuropsychological results in pediatric patients with epilepsy surgery in the parietal cortex. *Epilepsia* **49**, 700–704.

Gleissner, U., Sassen, R., Schramm, J., Elger, C.E. & Helmstaedter, C. (2005): Greater functional recovery after temporal lobe epilepsy surgery in children. *Brain* **128**, 2822–2829.

Guerrini, R. (2006): Epilepsy in children. *Lancet* **367**, 499–524.

Helmstaedter, C. & Kurthen, M. (2001): Memory and epilepsy: characteristics, course, and influence of drugs and surgery. *Curr. Opin. Neurol.* **14**, 211–216.

Hernandez, M.T., Sauerwein, H.C., Jambaqué, I., et al. (2003): Attention, memory, and behavioral adjustment in children with frontal lobe epilepsy. *Epilepsy Behav.* **4**, 522–536.

Jambaqué, I. & Dulac, O. (1989): Reversible frontal syndrome and epilepsy in a 8-year-old boy. *Arch. Fr. Pediatr.* **46**, 525–529.

Jonas, R., Nguyen, S., Hu, B., et al. (2004): Cerebral hemispherectomy: hospital course, seizure, developmental, language, and motor outcomes. *Neurology* **62**, 1712–1721.

Korkman, M., Granstrom, M.L., Kantola-Sorsa, E., et al. (2005): Two-year follow-up of intelligence after paediatric epilepsy surgery. *Pediatric Neurol.* **33**, 173–178.

Lagae, L., Pawels, J., Monté, C.P, Verbelle, B. & Vervish, J. (2001): Frontal absences in children. *Eur. J. Paediatr. Neurol.* **5**, 243–251.

Lah, S. (2004): Neuropsychological outcome following focal cortical removal for intractable epilepsy in children. *Epilepsy Behav.* **5**, 804–817.

Lassonde, M., Sauerwein, H.C., Jambaqué, I., Smith, M.L. & Helmstaeder, C. (2000): Neuropsychology of childhood epilepsy: pre and post surgical assessment. *Epileptic Disord.* **2**, 3–12.

Lee, Y.J., Kang, H.C., Lee, J.S., et al. (2010): Resective pediatric epilepsy surgery in Lennox-Gastaut syndrome. *Pediatrics.* **125**, 58–65.

Lendt, M., Gleissner, U., Helmstaedter, C., Sassen, R., Clusmann, H. & Elger, C.E. (2002): Neuropsychological outcome in children after frontal lobe epilepsy surgery. *Epilepsy Behav.* **3**, 51–59.

Lendt, M., Helmstaedter, C., Kuczaty, S., Schramm, J. & Elger, C.E. (2000): Behavioural disorders in children with epilepsy: early improvment after surgery. *Neurol. Neurosurg. Psych.* **69**, 739–744.

Loddenkeper, T., Holland, K.D., Stanford, L.D., Kotagal, P., Bingaman, W. & Wyllie, E. (2007): Developmental outcome after epilepsy surgery in infancy. *Pediatrics* **119**, 930–935.

McLellan, A. (2005): Psychopathology in children with epilepsy before and after temporal resection. *Dev. Med. Child Neurol.* **47**, 666–672.

Mabbot, D.J. & Smith, M.L. (2003). Memory in children with temporal or extra-temporal excision. *Neuropsychologia* **41**, 995–1007.

Meekes, J., Braams, O., Braun, P.J., Jennekens-Schinkel, A. & van Nieuwenhuizen, O; Dutch Collaborative Epilepsy Surgery Programme (DuCESP). (2013): Verbal memory after epilepsy surgery in childhood. *Epilepsy Res.* **107**, 146–155.

Mega, M.S., Cummings, J.L., Salloway, S. & Malloy, P. (1997): The limbic system: an anatomic, phylogenetic and clinical perspective. *J. Neuropsych. Clin. Neurosci.* **6**, 428–442.

Miranda, C. & Smith, M.L. (2001): Predictor of intelligence after temporal lobectomy in children with epilepsy. *Epilepsy Behav.* **2**, 13–19.

Nolan, M.A., Redoblado, M.A., Lah, S., et al. (2004): Memory function in childhood epilepsy syndromes. *J. Paed. Child Health.* **40**, 20–70.

Obeid, M., Willie, E., Rahi, A.C. & Mikati, M.A. (2009): Approach to pediatric epilepsy surgery: State of the art, Part I: General principles and presurgical workup. *Eur. J. Pediatr. Neurol.* **13**, 102–114.

Ounsted, C. (1969): Aggression and epilepsy rage in children with temporal lobe epilepsy. *J. Psychosom. Res.* **13**, 237–242.

Prévost, J., Lortie, A., Nguyen, D., Lassonde, M. & Carmant, L. (2006) Non-lesional frontal lobe epilepsy of childhood: clinical presentation, response to treatment and comorbidity. *Epilepsia* **47**, 2199–2201.

Pulsifer, M.B., Brandt, J., Salorio, C.F., Vining, E.P., Carson, B.S. & Freeman, J.M. (2004): The cognitive outcome of hemispherectomy in 71 children. *Epilepsia* **45**, 243–254.

Ramantani, G., Kadish, N.E., Strolb, K., *et al.* (2013): Seizure and cognitive outcomes of epilepsy surgery in infancy and early childhood. *Eur. J. Paed. Neur.* **17**, 498–506.

Rausch, R. (1991): Effects of temporal lobe surgery on behavior. *Adv. Neurol.* **55**, 279–292.

Riva, D., Avanzini, G., Franceschetti, S., *et al.* (2005): Unilateral frontal lobe epilepsy affects executive functions in children. *Neurol. Sci.* **26**, 263–270.

Riva, D., Saletti, V., Nichelli, F. & Bulgheroni, S. (2002): Neuropsychological effects of frontal lobe epilepsy in children. *J. Child Neurol.* **17**, 661–667.

Siegel, A.M. (2003): Parietal lobe epilepsy. *Adv. Neurol.* **93**, 335–345.

Skirrow, C., Cross, J.H., Cormack, F., Harkness, W., Varga-Khadem, F. & Baldeweg, T. (2011): Long-term Intellectual outcome after temporal lobe surgery in childhood. *Neurology* **76**, 1330–1337.

Smith, M.L., Elliot, I.M. & Lach, L. (2004): Cognitive, psychosocial, and family function one year after pediatric epilepsy surgery. *Epilepsia* **45**, 650–660.

Spencer, S. & Huh, L. (2008): Outcomes of epilepsy surgery in adults and children. *Lancet Neurol.* **7**, 525–537.

Sumer, D.B., Atik, L., Unal, A., Emure, U. & Atasoy, H.T. (2007): Frontal lobe epilepsy presented as ictal aggression. *Neurol. Sci.* **28**, 48–51.

Téllez-Zenteno, J.F., Dhar, R., Hernandez-Ronquillo, L. & Wiebe, S. (2007): Long-term outcomes in epilepsy surgery: antiepileptic drugs, mortality, cognitive and psychosocial aspects. *Brain* **130**, 334–345.

Van Schooneveld, M.M. & Braun, K.P. (2013): Cognitive outcome after epilepsy surgery in children. *Brain Dev.* **35**, 721–729.

Vasconcellos, E., Wyllie, E., Sullivan, S., Standford, L., Bulacio, J., Kotagal, P. & Bingaman, W. (2001): Mental retardation in pediatric candidates for epilepsy surgery: the role of early seizure onset. *Epilepsia* **42**, 268–274.

Viggedal, G., Kristjansdottir, R., Olsson, I., Rydenhag, B. & Uevbrant, P. (2012): Cognitive development from two to ten years after pediatric epilepsy surgery. *Epilepsy Behav.* **25**, 2–8.

Westerveld, M., Sass, K.J., Chelune, G.J., Hermann, B.P., Barr, W.B. & Loring, D.W. (2000): Temporal lobectomy in children: cognitive outcome. *J. Neurosurg.* **92**, 24–30.

Chapter 6

Cognitive and behavioural aspects of headache in children and adolescents

Umberto Balottin*°, Matteo Chiappedi*, Federica Galli*, Sara Gianfelice*, and Cristiano Termine[#]

*Child Neuropsychiatry Unit, C. Mondino National Neurological Institute, via Mondino 2, 27100 Pavia, Italy;
°Child Neuropsychiatry Unit, Dept. of Brain and Behavioural Sciences, University of Pavia, Italy;
[#]Child Neuropsychiatry Unit, Dept. of clinical and experimental medicine, University of Insubria Varese, Italy
umberto.balottin@unipv.it

Summary

Primary headaches in children and adolescents are defined according to the characteristics of pain and associated symptoms. There is stringent clinical evidence, however, that these disorders are associated with more complex alterations of the global functioning of the patient. Research regarding cognitive aspects is rather sparse and not consistent; the most significant (but not definitive) findings are a relative reduction of verbal academic intelligence and of short-term memory. On the other hand, based on psychological and behavioural aspects, there is a relatively high number of published papers, suggesting that psychopathological traits are significant factors linked to the course of the disease, such as frequency and severity of headache attacks. This leads to the conclusion that the study of psychological aspects (both psychopathological and psychosomatic factors) is of critical importance for the implementation of therapy. A two-fold neurological and psychiatric/psychological approach is needed for the assessment and treatment of these patients.

Introduction

The pathogenesis of tension-type headache and migraine are poorly defined, and this is relative to their diagnostic boundaries. Studies regarding cognitive function in children and adolescents with primary headache are sparse, whilst there is a large number of studies regarding behavioural and psychological aspects (Balottin *et al.*, 2013). However, it is clinically evident that these disorders cannot be understood and treated only as pain or neurological disorders, given the importance of the whole cognitive and behavioural profile of these children and adolescents.

Cognitive aspects

As already mentioned, this topic has been almost neglected in the scientific literature. In adults, despite the associations observed between migraine and structural brain lesions (*e.g.* white matter abnormalities), cognitive function does not appear to be affected by significant structural changes (Rist & Kurth, 2013), even if there is a lack of data regarding the effects of headache characteristics, such as the frequency of the attacks. Moreover, even the likely changes in cognitive functioning associated with non-migraine headache should be clarified with further studies.

A study by Palm-Meinders (2012), a 9-year follow-up involving 295 adult women with primary headache, showed the occurrence of signal alteration of deep white matter on MRI, with a higher incidence compared to the control group. The authors, however, did not find any significant cognitive differences between groups. On the other hand, Hagen and colleagues (2014), in a prospective study involving 51,323 subjects, found an odds ratio of 2.2 for the risk of developing vascular dementia (and an odds ratio of 2.0 for any kind of dementia) in the group of patients with headache of any kind. Studies examining children and adolescents are even less consistent.

A multicentre controlled trial by Parisi and collaborators (2010) involved 63 children with migraine, 19 with tension-type headache, and 79 without headache. These authors found significant difference in IQ (measured with the Italian version of the Weschler Intelligence Scale for Childhood-Revised (WISC-III); the control group had an average IQ of 115, dropping to 110 and 108 in children with tension-type headache and migraine, respectively. Although average IQ and sub-scores were in the normal range for all groups of patients, the statistically significant difference was due to the lower verbal intelligence found in subjects with headache. It is worth noting that the only significant independent variable predicting these differences was the frequency of headache attacks.

Esposito and colleagues (2012) compared two groups of children: 75 with migraine without aura and 72 with tension-type headache, including a control group of 137 children. The authors showed no significant differences in terms of IQ, but a higher performance IQ in children with tension-type headache (average value: 101.4) compared to the control group (average value: 95), who had, in turn, a higher performance IQ compared to children with migraine (average value: 92.7), although the difference was not statistically significant. It is also worth noting that this study evidenced a reduction of perceptual organization which was significant only for children with migraine (91.4 *versus* 96.6), while the verbal IQ was significantly reduced only in the group of children with tension-type headache (98.6 *versus* 105.3).

In another controlled study conducted in São Paulo by Moutran and collaborators (2011), 30 children and adolescents with migraine were compared with 30 control subjects. The authors found a significantly lower average IQ in the migraine group (102.8 *versus* 113.7); both the verbal (102.4 *versus* 113.1) and performance (102.8 *versus* 112.2) IQs were significantly different. Since the WISC-III was used in this study, the authors performed a comparison between the different factorial indexes which can be obtained by this version of the Weschler Intelligence Scale for Children; they found a nearly significant reduction of verbal comprehension (113.3 *versus* 112.0) and a significant reduction of perceptual organization (110.4 *versus* 101.7), freedom from distractibility (110.1 *versus* 98.5), and processing speed (11.6 *versus* 104.2).

Riva and collaborators (2012) studied 62 children with different forms of primary headache compared to 52 controls. Using the Conners' Continuous Performance Test, these authors witnessed no significant differences in the pattern of attention between children with different forms of headache. However, the authors showed shorter reaction times and an increase in the number of commission errors in children with migraine compared to the control group; this was interpreted to be suggestive of an impulsive response style in children with migraine.

More recently, Genizi (2013), in a medical centre in Haifa, retrospectively reviewed medical records of 243 children and adolescents with primary headache and found a significantly higher prevalence of ADHD (attention deficit hyperactivity disorder) and learning disabilities. In contrast, another study on primary headache did not find any association both with ADHD overall and the inattention component, even though a significant association had been found with the hyperactive-impulsive component of ADHD (Arruda, 2010). Parisi and colleagues (2012) compared patients with benign epilepsy with centro-temporal spikes (BECTS) to patients with this epileptic disorder and migraine as well as patients with migraine and centro-temporal spikes (CTS). They found no significant differences in terms of IQ, however, using a more detailed assessment (the NEPSY-II), a difference was found in both groups with migraine with regards to reduced long-term verbal memory.

Taken as a whole, these data confirm that, in children and adolescents with headache, the average IQ is in the normal range; the comparisons with control groups showed no consistent differences, but indicate the possibility of a complex frame of neuropsychological vulnerabilities involving visuo-perceptual skills, attention, verbal memory, and processing speed. As in adults, the potential role of headache characteristics (*e.g.* the frequency of attacks) should be addressed in further studies.

Behavioural aspects

Many studies have analyzed the behavioural aspects of children and adolescents suffering from headache. Using stringent criteria, in terms of methodological relevance, less than 20 reports where considered relevant: seven population-based studies, five controlled studies, two systematic reviews, and three meta-analyses, *i.e.* a significant number of methodologically-sound papers have been published, enough to provide data for a meta-analysis.

Taken as a whole, reports appear to converge, demonstrating that a relevant and clinically significant level of psychopathological aspects is found in children and adolescents with primary headache.

Lanzi and colleagues (1983, 1988) administered the Rorschach test to 15 subjects who had migraine with aura, 15 subjects who had migraine without aura, and 15 subjects who had chronic daily headache, and compared their results with those obtained from 29 control subjects. They reported the presence of highly relevant and significant personality characteristics which were distinguishing features of subjects with or without headache, with only subtle differences among the different forms of headache. In detail, subjects with headache more often gave responses involving the use of white space and popular responses, *i.e.* responses which are most commonly given from an epidemiological point of view. Moreover, subjects with headache more often presented a kinesthetic shock (*i.e.* a lack of human, or human-like movement) and specific responses characterized by static movement. On the other hand, there was a lower number of responses involving movement of any kind and a lower level of formal accuracy (*i.e.* the percentage of responses of good formal level or F+). These authors demonstrated that subjects with headache show a low level of empathy and introspective ability (also referred to as 'insight'); these mechanisms, in turn, determine a high degree of conformity, a tendency to think and act as others through a mechanism of hyper-adaptation. In addition, a low level of emotional control and a strong tendency to oppositional and defiant functioning seem to emerge from the detailed study of response protocols. This study is interesting because it combines acceptable methodological rigor (use of a standardized and quantified test) and the use of a specific test for personality characteristics of adolescents.

A follow-up study by Guidetti and colleagues (1998) confirmed the association between primary headache, depression, and anxiety, also providing evidence of the causal value of anxiety and depression in predicting a negative outcome for headache. Dilsaver and collaborators (2009) reported a controlled study performed on a clinical Latin American population and offered significant data and elements to support the existence of a privileged link between migraine and depression in adolescents (odds ratio: 5.98).

Population-based studies are consistent in confirming the relationship between psychopathology and recurrent headaches in children and adolescents. Egger and colleagues (1999) confirmed the association between anxiety disorders and headache and other pain disorders in girls. Ando and collaborators (2013) studied more than 18,000 adolescents and reported a significant association between the number of body parts affected by pain (including headache) and the degree of mental health impairment. Arruda and Bigal (2012), in a relevant population study of 1,850 adolescents, found a significant association between internalizing symptoms and primary headaches. This was confirmed by the increased prevalence of psychopathological symptoms (especially emotional disorders and hyperactivity and/or attention deficit) seen in a population of 18,000 adolescents with headache (Milde-Busch *et al.,* 2010).

Finally, recent meta-analytic studies have confirmed the presence of significant psychopathological comorbidity in children and adolescents with recurrent idiopathic headache (both migraine and tension-type).

A meta-analysis by Pinquart and Shen (2011a) integrated results from 332 published studies to assess the role of anxiety in children and adolescents with chronic physical illnesses. They found significantly higher levels of anxiety in subjects with any of these disorders; primary headaches were among the single disorders with the highest anxiety level compared to controls (Cohen's d = 0.42; average for all disorders: Cohen's d = 0.18).

Balottin and colleagues (2013) performed a meta-analysis and selected 10 studies on the basis of a widely used psychodiagnostic tool (the Child Behavior Checklist [CBCL]) and by applying rigorous criteria; the studies were compared in a meta-analysis in order to evaluate the presence of internalizing (mainly anxiety and depression) and externalizing (mainly behavioural problems) symptoms in different types of headache (also *versus* healthy controls). Patients with migraine showed more psychopathological symptoms than healthy controls. Patients with tension-type headache (TTH) also exhibited more psychopathology than controls, although the difference was more marked for internalizing disorders. Finally, no differences emerged between migraine and TTH.

Another meta-analysis by Pinquart and Shen (2011b) integrated results from 569 published studies to explore the risk of emotional and behavioural problems in children and adolescents with chronic physical illnesses. They found higher levels of internalizing (Hedge's g = 0.47), externalizing (Hedge's g = 0.22), and total behavioural problems (Hedge's g = 0.42) in these patients; primary headaches were among the disorders with the greatest increase in internalizing (Hedge's g = 0.77), externalizing (Hedge's g = 0.36), and total behavioural problems (Hedge's g = 0.75).

Balottin and colleagues (2004, 2005) showed a significant association between important life events and the onset of headache and isolated attacks in children under 6 years of age. Stress has been confirmed as the main risk factor for headache in adolescents, as shown for the lack of physical exercise, coffee use, and alcohol abuse (Milde-Busch *et al.*, 2012). Finally, Tietjen and collaborators (2010) showed the importance of maltreatment and emotional abuse of children as risk factors for developing headache in adolescence and adult age.

Conclusions

Regarding cognitive aspects, the existing literature is not consistent and the presence and specific characterization of cognitive deficits in children and adolescents with primary headaches is still uncertain and debated. The most convincing evidence is derived from academic intelligence measured using the Weschler's intelligence scales; although the average IQs tend to fall in the normal range, they are usually significantly lower than those of controls and this is especially true for the verbal component of intelligence. Short-term memory is often found to be reduced in patients with headache (Moutran *et al.*, 2011). Preliminary findings also suggest the existence of a possible correlation between seizure frequency and cognitive damage in patients with both headache and epilepsy (including the so-called 'benign' forms), but these data need to be replicated in larger samples and in longitudinal studies.

Regarding behavioural and psychopathological aspects, the majority of children and adolescents with migraine do not present with any disorder which may be diagnosed according to commonly used self-report questionnaires or semi-structured clinical interviews (Balottin *et al.*, 2011). However, when population data, controlled studies, and meta-analysis are taken into account, there is strong evidence that psychopathological disorders are a significant risk factor for primary headache in children and adolescents. Among these disorders, a major role is probably played by internalizing disorders, such as depression, anxiety, and stress-related disturbances. It is also worth noting that psychological and psycho-behavioural techniques have been demonstrated to be the most effective treatments for reducing severity and frequency of headache attacks (Eccleston *et al.*, 2012).

To conclude, cognitive aspects of primary headaches in children and adolescent need to be further studied, especially to explore the presence of cognitive damage related to headache attacks and the possible association with ADHD and/or specific learning disorders, which could have relevant consequences on academic achievement. As for psychopathological and behavioural aspects, there are convincing data supporting the presence of a psychiatric component with a relevant role in the pathogenesis of primary headaches. For the clinical diagnostic and therapeutic approach, it is important to consider psychopathological and behavioural aspects, and this should be based on both neurological and psychiatric/psychological competences.

Conflicts of interest: none.

References

Ando, S., Yamasaki, S., Shimodera, S., *et al.* (2013): A greater number of somatic pain sites is associated with poor mental health in adolescents: a cross-sectional study. *BMC Psychiatry* **13**, 30.

Arruda, M.A. & Bigal, M.E. (2012): Behavioral and emotional symptoms and primary headaches in children: a population-based study. *Cephalalgia* **32**, 1093–1100.

Arruda, M.A., Guidetti, V., Galli, F., Albuquerque, R.C. & Bigal, M.E. (2010): Migraine, tension-type headache, and attention-deficit/hyperactivity disorder in childhood: a population-based study. *Postgrad. Med.* **122,** 18–26.

Balottin, U., Nicoli, F., Pitillo, G., Ferrari-Ginevra, O., Borgatti, R. & Lanzi, G. (2004): Migraine and tension headache in children under 6 years of age. *Eur. J. Pain* **8,** 307–314.

Balottin, U., Termine, C., Nicoli, F., Quadrelli, M., Ferrari-Ginevra, O. & Lanzi, G. (2005): Idiopathic headache in children under 6 years of age: a follow-up study. *Headache* **45,** 705–715.

Balottin, U., Chiappedi, M., Rossi, M., Termine, C. & Nappi, G. (2011): Childhood and adolescent migraine: a neuropsychiatric disorder? *Med. Hypotheses* **76,** 778–781.

Balottin, U., Fusar Poli, P., Termine, C., Molteni, S. & Galli, F. (2013): Psychopathological symptoms in child and adolescent migraine and tension-type headache: a meta-analysis. *Cephalalgia* **33,** 112–122.

Dilsaver, S.C., Benazzi, F., Oedegaard, K.J., Fasmer, O.B., Akiskal, K.K. & Akiskal, H.S. (2009): Migraine in affectively ill Mexican adolescents. *World Psychiatry* **8,** 37–39.

Eccleston, C., Palermo, T.M., de C Williams, A.C., *et al.* (2012): Psychological therapies for the management of chronic and recurrent pain in children and adolescents. *Cochrane Database Syst. Rev.* **12,** 12.

Egger, H.L., Costello, E.J., Erkanli, A. & Angold, A. (1999): Somatic complaints and psychopathology in children and adolescents: stomach aches, musculoskeletal pains, and headaches. *J. Am. Acad. Child Adolesc. Psychiatry* **38**: 852–860.

Esposito, M., Pascotto, A., Gallai, B., *et al.* (2012): Can headache impair intellectual abilities in children? An observational study. *Neuropsychiatr. Dis. Treat.* **8,** 509–513.

Genizi, J., Gordon, S., Kerem, N.C., Srugo, I., Shahar, E. & Ravid, S. (2013): Primary headaches, attention deficit disorder and learning disabilities in children and adolescents. *J. Headache Pain* **27,** 54.

Guidetti, V., Galli, F., Fabrizi, P., *et al.* (1998): Headache and psychiatric comorbidity: clinical aspects and outcome in an 8-year follow-up study. *Cephalalgia* **18,** 455–462.

Hagen, K., Stordal, E., Linde, M., Steiner, T.J., Zwart, J.A. & Stovner, L.J. (2014): Headache as a risk factor for dementia: a prospective population-based study. *Cephalalgia* **34,** 327–335.

Lanzi, G., Balottin, U., Gamba, N. & Fazzi, E. (1983): Psychological aspects of migraine in childhood. *Cephalalgia* **3,** 218–220.

Lanzi, G., Balottin, U., Borgatti, R., Guderzo, M. & Scarabello, E. (1988): Different forms of migraine in childhood and adolescence: notes on personality traits. *Headache* **28,** 618–622.

Milde-Busch, A., Boneberger, A., Heinrich, S., *et al.* (2010): Higher prevalence of psychopathological symptoms in adolescents with headache. A population-based cross-sectional study. *Headache* **50,** 738–748.

Milde-Busch, A., Straube, A., Heinen, F. & von Kries, R. (2012): Identified risk factors and adolescents' beliefs about triggers for headaches: results from a cross-sectional study. *J. Headache Pain.* **13**(8), 639–643.

Moutran, A.R., Villa, T.R., Diaz, L.A., *et al.* (2011): Migraine and cognition in children: a controlled study. *Arq. Neuropsiquiatr.* **69,** 192–195.

Palm-Meinders, I.H., Koppen, H., Terwindt, G.M., *et al.* (2012): Structural brain changes in migraine. *JAMA* **308,** 1889–1897.

Parisi, P., Verrotti, A., Paolino, M.C., *et al.* (2010): Headache and cognitive profile in children: a cross-sectional controlled study. *J. Headache Pain* **11**: 45–51.

Parisi, P., Matricardi, S., Tozzi, E., Sechi, E., Martini, C. & Verrotti, A. (2012): Benign epilepsy of childhood with centro-temporal spikes (BECTS) *versus* migraine: a neuropsychological assessment. *Childs Nerv. Syst.* **28,** 2129–2135.

Pinquart, M. & Shen, Y. (2011a): Anxiety in children and adolescents with chronic physical illnesses: a meta-analysis. *Acta. Paediatr.* **100,** 1069–1076.

Pinquart, M. & Shen, Y. (2011b): Behavior problems in children and adolescents with chronic physical illness: a meta-analysis. *J. Pediatr. Psychol.* **36,** 1003–1016.

Rist, P.M. & Kurth, T. (2013): Migraine and cognitive decline: a topical review. *Headache* **53,** 589–598.

Riva, D., Usilla, A., Aggio, F., Vago, C., Treccani, C. & Bulgheroni, S. (2012): Attention in children and adolescents with headache. *Headache* **52,** 374–384.

Tietjen, G.E., Brandes, J.L., Peterlin, B.L., *et al.* (2010): Childhood maltreatment and migraine (part II). Emotional abuse as a risk factor for headache chronification. *Headache* **50,** 32–41.

Malformations and tumours

Chapter 7

Spina bifida: brain and neurobehavioural outcomes

Jack M. Fletcher*, Jennifer J. Juranek° and Maureen Dennis[#]

* Dept. of Psychology, Texas Institute for Measurement, Evaluation, and Statistics, University of Houston, 4811 Calhoun, Room 488, Houston, TX 77204-6062, USA;
° Dept. of Paediatrics, University of Texas Health Science Center at Houston, Houston, TX, USA;
[#] Program in Neurosciences and Mental Health, The Hospital for Sick Children, Toronto, Ontario, Canada
jack.fletcher@times.uh.edu

Summary

Neurobehavioural outcomes in spina bifida myelomeningocele (SBM) are variable, although there is a modal profile. This paper reviews the physical and neural phenotypes associated with SBM, the pattern of neurobehavioural outcomes, and their relations. In addition to the level of spinal lesion, SBM is associated with distinctive brain malformations involving the cerebellum, midbrain, and corpus callosum that are directly related to core deficits in timing, attention, and movement. In addition, there are secondary effects of hydrocephalus and its treatment, and the psychosocial environment. The core deficits lead to strengths in associative learning and weaknesses in assembled learning and integrative processes. Comprehensive early interventions that take advantage of the modal profile and variations around it are essential for people with SBM.

Introduction

Spina bifida, a neurogenetic disorder, is the most common birth defect affecting the central nervous system (CNS) in the world compatible with survival (Liptak, 2013). A neural tube defect, spina bifida historically has been identified at birth because of the characteristic spinal dysraphism that gives the disorder its name ('split spine'). Presently, spina bifida is often identified before birth primarily through ultrasonography and alpha fetoprotein testing (Copp *et al.*, 2013). The most common form of spina bifida, myelomeningocele, is an open defect with the spinal cord and meninges protruding anywhere along the spinal column (Detrait *et al.*, 2005). Representing 90 per cent of all spina bifida cases, it is the only form of spina bifida that is reliably associated with malformations of the brain and hydrocephalus. Other forms of spina bifida, such as meningocele and lipoma, are 'closed' defects that have an infrequent association with brain dysmorphology, although orthopaedic and urological complications are frequent. In the remainder of this chapter, discussion will be restricted to spina bifida myelomeningocele (SBM) because of the association with brain anomalies and neuropsychological difficulties related to these anomalies.

Because of its complexity, the assessment and treatment of SBM begins before birth and through adulthood, involving multiple disciplines. The difficulties with assessment and treatment of SBM stem from its multiple sources of phenotypic variability: physical, neurological, and neuropsychological. In this chapter, we focus on findings from a program of research attempting genetic, neuroimaging, and neuropsychological studies of a common cohort of children and adults with SBM in Houston and Toronto that began in 1998, with data collection through 2010 (Fletcher et al., 2004).

Physical phenotype

Few children with any form of spina bifida are spared problems with urological functions and ambulation, although they may not be less severe in cases that are not open defects or with sacral level spinal lesions; most children with upper level (thoracic and above) spinal lesions are paraplegic. Generally, the higher the spinal dysraphism, the greater the orthopaedic impairment. Higher level defects are also associated both with greater severity of brain malformations and poorer cognitive and motor outcomes, most likely because of greater impairment in brain structure (Fletcher et al., 2005). Lesion level also accounts for genetic heterogeneity, as does ethnicity and socioeconomic status (Au et al., 2010). In particular, spinal lesions at the thoracic level and above are most deleterious not only in terms of lower extremity difficulties, but also general cognitive functioning. These upper level defects occur more frequently in Hispanics than non-Hispanics, which is related to the heritability of SBM (Au et al., 2010).

Fig. 1 depicts the relation of lesion level with gross motor functions, fine motor functions, and IQ. The gross motor difficulties are significant across the range of spinal lesion levels, but are clearly more severe in thoracic level spinal lesions. Fine motor skills are less impaired, but more impaired than in lumbar and sacral lesions. IQ scores are above the range (on average) associated with intellectual deficiency (IQ < 70) even in the thoracic group, but the thoracic group performs well below those with lumbar and sacral lesions. It is important to recognize that lesion level *per se* does not cause the IQ differences; rather, higher level lesions have greater brain dysmorphology that is likely related to poorer outcomes.

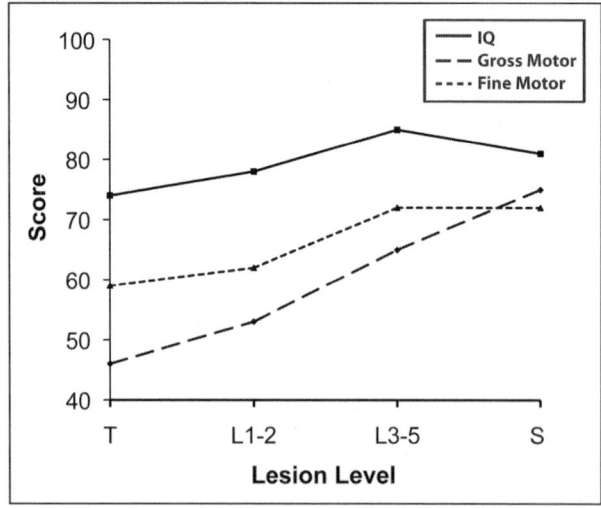

Fig. 1. Relation of spinal lesion level and gross motor functions, fine motor functions, and IQ. There is a pattern of increasing poor performance in all three domains with thoracic level spinal lesions.

Brain

The brain of a person with SBM is dysmorphic and associated with malformations of the hindbrain that lead to a spectrum of anomalies represented as the Chiari II malformation, with mechanical effects on the cerebellum and midbrain from development of these structures in a small posterior fossa. The Chiari II malformation occurs in over 90 per cent of people with SBM. In addition to downward herniation of the cerebellum into the foramen of Monro, there are often midbrain anomalies, with the tectum achieving a beaked appearance in over half those with SBM (Barkovich & Raybaud, 2012).

Hypogenesis (partial absence) and hypoplasia (thinning) of the corpus callosum are also common, usually affecting the posterior body, splenium, and the rostrum. Although most people with SBM have abnormalities of the corpus callosum, the range of anomaly is broad (Hannay et al., 2009). Fig. 2 depicts a series of midsagittal MRIs showing the Chiari malformation, hypogenesis and hypoplasia of the corpus callosum, and tectal beaking.

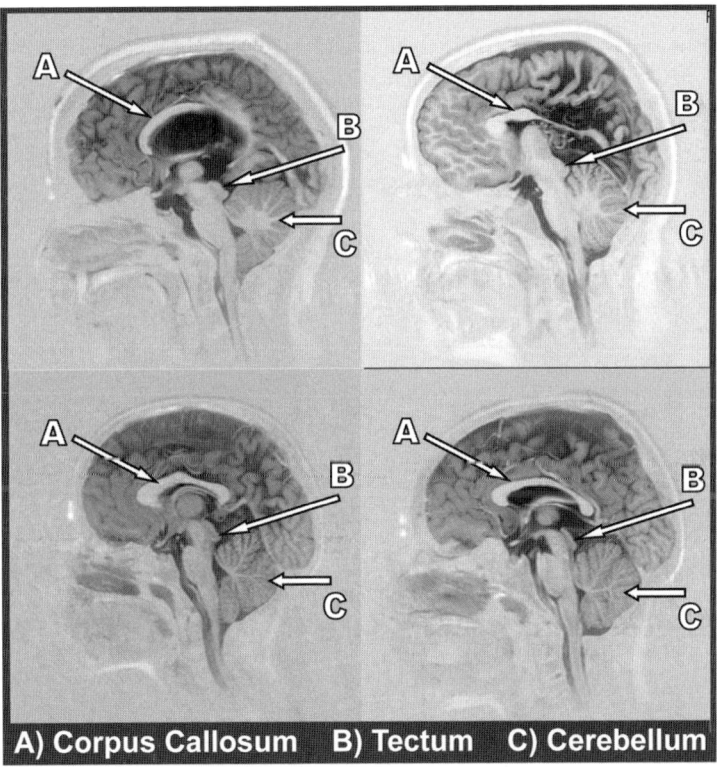

Fig. 2. Four midsagittal MRI slices illustrating the variability in brain dysmorphology in spina bifida myelomeningocele, all shunted for hydrocephalus. In each figure, A represents the corpus callosum; B represents the tectum; and C represents the cerebellum. The upper left MRI slice shows significant dilation of the lateral ventricles, a corpus callosum that is thinned by hydrocephalus, and a malformed, downwardly shifted cerebellum consistent with a moderate Chiari II malformation. The lower left shows a corpus callosum that is mildly thinned in the splenium, no ventricular dilation, a slightly beaked tectum, and a mild Chiari II malformation. In the upper right panel, the patient shows residual hydrocephalus, significant hypogenesis of the splenium and posterior body of the corpus callosum, tectal beaking, and a significant Chiari II malformation. The lower right panel shows lateral ventricle dilation less severe than the upper left panel, hypogenesis of the rostrum and thinning of the posterior corpus callosum, no tectal beaking, and a significant Chiari II malformation.

Hydrocephalus is a common sequel of the Chiari II malformation, which obstructs the flow of cerebrospinal fluid at the level of the fourth ventricle. Fig. 2 shows varying degrees of ventricular dilation in the four people with SBM, all of whom have been shunted for hydrocephalus. Some form of ventriculomegaly is usually present, often requiring shunting with a vetriculoperitoneal shunt or endoscopic third ventriculostomy. Although at one time it was routine to shunt when the spinal lesion was repaired at birth, many neurosurgical centres monitor the child's development and insert shunts later in development when the hydrocephalus appears to be interfering with development (Bowman & McLone, 2010).

Quantitative assessments of MRI show variations in cortical development that represent atypical organization (Juranek & Salman, 2010). Cerebral volumes show reductions of grey and white matter in the cerebrum, excluding the frontal lobes, which show higher grey matter compared to typically developing children (Juranek et al., 2008). Cerebellar volumes are lower in SBM than controls in a stepwise manner in which upper level spinal lesions are associated with greater reductions than lower level lesions (Fletcher et al., 2005). The atypical organization of the cerebellum, however, is not linear, but represents quantitative shifts in which the anterior cerebellum is larger, the posterior-inferior regions are smaller, and there is no difference in the corpus medullare (Juranek et al., 2010). In the cortex, the frontal, superior parietal, and occipital regions are thicker, while inferior parietal and temporal regions are thinner (Juranek et al., 2008; Treble et al., 2012).

There are also variations in cortical volumes in which some parts are too large and some are too small. This variation is depicted in Fig. 3. Like Williams syndrome (Meda et al., 2012)

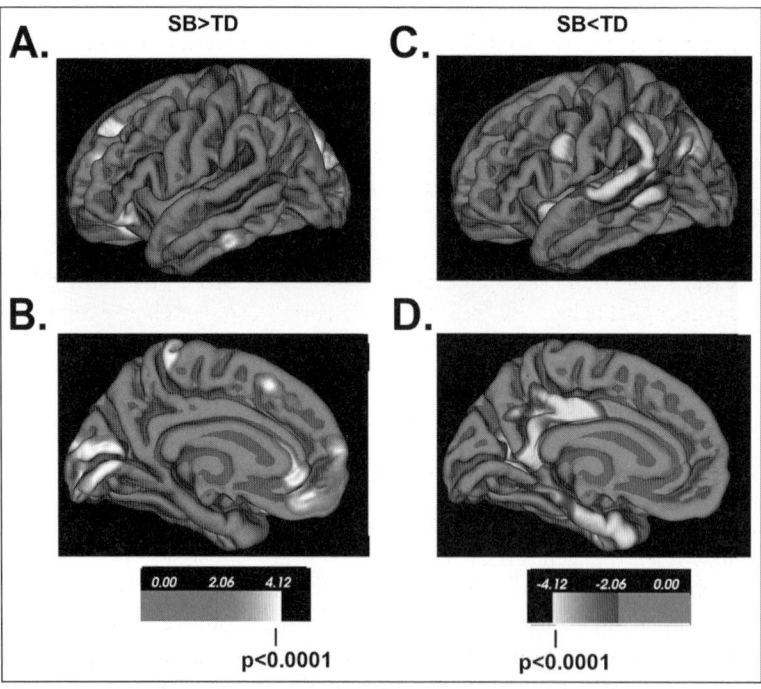

Fig. 3. Differences in cortical thickness between individuals with SBM and a comparison group of typically-developing (TD) study participants. Lighter colors indicate cortical thickness is greater in the SBM group relative to the TD group; darker colors indicate cortical thickness is reduced in the SBM group relative to the TD group. In frontal regions, the SBM group exhibits increased cortical thickness bilaterally in the inferior frontal, middle frontal, medial orbitofrontal, rostral anterior cingulate, and superior frontal regions. Cortical thinning is apparent in bilateral inferior parietal and posterior temporal areas.

many people with SBM have 'fat' frontal lobes and thinning in the posterior regions, but this pattern is not uniform or comparable in other regions across disorders (*e.g.* basal ganglia). Assessments of gyral development in SBM also show regional differences, with higher gyrification (increased cortical folding) in the lateral frontal, inferior parietal, and posterior temporal regions. Gyrification is lower in the inferior frontal lobe and the medial surface of the parietal and temporal lobes (Treble *et al.*, 2012).

The basal ganglia and related subcortical structures are visibly normal on radiological review in SBM (Ware *et al.*, 2014). On quantitative macrostructural assessment, the hippocampus, but not the amygdala, is reduced in volume (Treble-Barna *et al.*, 2015; Ware *et al.*, 2014). The putamen is enlarged. Diffusion tensor imaging of white matter structures shows that the integrity of the long association fibre tracts connecting posterior and anterior brain regions is consistently reduced relative to controls (Hasan *et al.*, 2008a; Ou *et al.*, 2011). Reduced integrity has also been shown in the genu of the corpus callosum, but not in the anterior commissure (Herweh *et al.*, 2009). Using the midbrain as a seed point in an analysis of tectal beaking, Williams and colleagues (2013) reported that posterior pathways showed greater reduction in white matter integrity than frontal pathways, especially in people with SBM and tectal beaking.

These studies show that the cerebrum of people with SBM is atypically organized on an anterior to posterior gradient. Volumetric studies show that some specific structures are reduced in volume (hippocampus), while others are enlarged relative to controls (putamen). In addition, there are specific malformations involving the cerebellum, midbrain, and corpus callosum that are associated with aberrant connectivity. At a microstructural level, connectivity and integrity of specific brain regions are reduced, but not in a uniform direction. For example, the caudate shows increased fractional anisotropy that may be related to a failure of pruning that leads to excessive dendritic branching (Hasan *et al.*, 2008b; Ware *et al.*, 2014).

The mechanical effects of hydrocephalus contribute to these patterns of atypical organization. Hydrocephalus represents ventricular expansion that leads to destruction of periventricular white matter (Del Bigio, 2010). This expansion also affects the regional distribution of white and grey matter, with cortical thickness lower along the lateral and third ventricles. However, the fact that the corpus callosum is hypogenetic in about half of children with SBM cannot be explained by hydrocephalus because the ends of the corpus callosum have simply not developed (Barkovich & Raybaud, 2012). A major question involves the consequences of this atypical organization for neuropsychological functions.

Relations of brain and neurobehavioural outcomes

Not surprisingly, given these complexities, cognitive and psychosocial outcomes are variable in SBM. The modal neuropsychological phenotype (Dennis & Barnes, 2010) involves the preservation of grammar and vocabulary, but with poor pragmatics and comprehension, and hypersociality, good word reading, but poor reading comprehension and mathematics. Intellectual disabilities are infrequent, occurring primarily in relation to upper level spinal lesions and poverty. Social adjustment difficulties emerge as children age, but children with SBM have low social anxiety (Holmbeck *et al.*, 2006). Problems in school are common because of learning and attention difficulties. In one large cohort, one-third of children had elevated parent ratings of ADHD behaviour, largely on the inattentive scale (Burmeister *et al.*, 2005). While only 3 per cent had word decoding problems, 26 per cent had problems in mathematics and another 23 per cent had both difficulties in mathematics and reading decoding (Fletcher *et al.*, 2005). These characteristics persist in adults, with many with spina bifida under-employed relative to literacy and IQ. In one study of adult outcomes, functional skills in mathematics were the best predictor of independent living (Hetherington *et al.*, 2006).

These features vary with the individual in a principled manner reflecting the severity of congenital malformations, regional brain development, and hydrocephalus. Not every individual with SBM shows the modal pattern, which also varies according to environmental patterns, treatment of hydrocephalus, ethnicity, and genetic factors (Dennis *et al.*, 2006). At this point, the capacity to assess the brain and relate these assessments to neuropsychological outcomes shows that the variation is predictable and principled. From the measurements of atypical organization summarized above, specific correlates can be described.

Cerebellum

A contemporary perspective on the cerebellum focuses on its role in harmonizing movement, especially the precision of fine motor movements, which includes rhythmicity and timing. Adults and children who are impaired in cerebellar functions show impairment in perceptual and motor timing, and rhythm discrimination and production. These same difficulties have been demonstrated in children with SBM (Dennis *et al.*, 2010). The perceptual and motor deficits are correlated with cerebellar volumes. In addition, on motor learning tasks, children with SBM are impaired in performance, but not in adaptation. As they perform a learning task, their capacity to benefit from repetition (procedural learning) is similar to controls, even though their performance is slower and poorer in quality (Edelstein *et al.*, 2004). Because procedural learning is mediated by frontal striatal regions, this pattern implies that motor learning mediated by the basal ganglia may be relatively intact. These patterns likely represent specific effects of the cerebellar malformation that is part of the Chiari II malformation (Dennis *et al.*, 2010).

Corpus callosum

The corpus callosum is responsible for connecting the two hemispheres, supporting interhemispheric communication and the integration of information. Children with hypogenesis of the corpus callosum show reduced auditory interhemispheric communication that is correlated with a measurement of the area of the splenium (Hannay *et al.*, 2009). Children with severe hypoplasia or hypogenesis have more difficulty understanding idioms and jokes, reflecting problems with abstraction, a high level skill requiring integration of information (Dennis & Barnes, 2010).

Midbrain

The beaking of the tectum is a specific marker for difficulties orienting and shifting attentional focus. These functions are viewed as a product of a posterior attention system involving the midbrain and parietal lobes that responds to salient features of the environment and is related to alertness and arousal. These attention functions are poorer in children with SBM who have tectal beaking. Connectivity from the midbrain is reduced in those with SBM and tectal beaking. Performance on covert orienting tasks is correlated with tectal beaking (Dennis *et al.*, 2005) and with tectal volume in SBM (Kulesz *et al.*, 2015). Interestingly, children with congenital hydrocephalus secondary to aqueductal stenosis do not show poorer performance than controls on covert attention tasks (Treble-Barna *et al.*, 2014) and perform significantly better than children with SBM and tectal beaking. In contrast, children with SBM are less impaired on attention tasks that require top-down regulatory processes associated with an anterior attention system mediated by frontal-striatal brain circuits. This is the system that is impaired in children with ADHD (Dennis et al., 2008). In one study, children with early hydrocephalus showed a different pattern on a test of attention persistence requiring sustained attention (Brewer et al., 2001). Children with SBM and ADHD had similarly impaired initial levels of slower response to this task than controls, but as the task progressed, children with ADHD performed even more poorly, but children with SBM stabilized. By the last parts of the task, their performance was similar to the controls.

Cortical thickness and thinning

An interesting question is whether the atypical patterns of cortical thickness and gyrification represent potential compensatory mechanisms in people with SBM. For example, a 'fatter' frontal lobe might be related to higher IQ scores. In fact, Treble and colleagues (2012) did not find evidence that these extreme deviations were associated with better outcomes. Rather, children at either extreme of cortical thickness or thinning tended to have lower IQ scores and better fine motor skills. Children closer to the normative values had better cognitive development.

Subcortical structures

The patterns of variability in subcortical structures are also related to variability in outcomes. Hasan and collaborators (2008b) reported lower correlations of IQ scores with increased fractional anisotropy of the caudate. Prospective memory is the ability to remember future intentions (i.e. remembering to remember), while episodic memory is a retrospective recall of specific events and learning. Treble-Barna and colleagues (2015) found that lower hippocampal (but not amygdala) volumes were associated with poorer prospective and episodic memory skills across the lifespan in children and adults with SBM.

Brain and cognition in SBM: what does it mean?

People with SBM have congenitally malformed brains and atypical brain organizations that lead to strengths and weaknesses in cognitive and motor outcomes. In examining both types of data, we have argued that there are three core impairments in SBM: timing, attention, and movement (Dennis et al., 2006). Timing is derived from the effects of SBM on the cerebellum; attention from the midbrain; and movement from the orthopaedic effects and the cerebellum. Core deficits are apparent early in development and persist. For example, Taylor and collaborators (2013) were able to identify attention orienting deficits in infants with SBM at six months of age using a task involving attending and orienting to a mobile.

Table 1. Strengths and weaknesses in cognitive domains for children and adults with spina bifida myelomeningocele

	Associative processing	Assembled processing
Domain	**Assets**	**Deficits**
Motor	Motor learning	Motor control
Perception	Face recognition	Spatial relations
Language	Vocabulary and grammar	Listening comprehension
Reading	Decoding	Comprehension
Mathematics	Fact retrieval	Algorithms
Behaviour	Sociability	Regulation

Core deficits can be exacerbated by the effects of hydrocephalus, which reduce neural connectivity and intensify timing and attention deficits. Core deficits also interact with the environment, with the modal profile emerging primarily in environments that are supportive of development, such as reduced poverty and psychosocial adversity. In such circumstances, a person with SBM will show strengths in cognitive processes that involve associative learning and weaknesses in learning that requires assembling and integration of memory. This, information that can be learned by repetition, memorization, repeated exposure, and other examples of associative earning are often relative strengths in SBM. In contrast, cognitive weaknesses involve content that must be integrated, summarized, or assembled. As Table 1 shows, these strengths are not specific to content domains, but occur within domains depending on whether learning is more associative or integrative. The likelihood of observing this modal profile is reduced if hydrocephalus is severe, there are treatment complications or secondary problems (*e.g.* brain infection), or in the face of psychosocial adversity.

Assessment and intervention

People with spina bifida require comprehensive assessments. They may require special schooling and rehabilitation, the services of an urologist and orthopaedist, neurosurgical intervention and follow-ups, and assistance with parenting and psychological adjustment. The assessments begin early in development and may include functional neurological and orthopaedic assessments, urological assessment, neurosurgical assessment, and neuropsychological assessments from a multi-disciplinary perspective (Fletcher *et al.*, 2008).

From a neuropsychological perspective, it is useful to understand the modal profile and attempt to identify it within content domains. The variability around the modal profile is significant and not simply captured by referring to problems with attention and executive function. Motor functions are important for overall adaptation. Attention problems are more likely to reflect problems with inattention and arousal that reflect lack of access to online self-regulatory processes as opposed to a disorder of disinhibition and self-regulation observed in many people with ADHD. A careful assessment of academic skills is needed, especially because of the common need for programming in reading comprehension, mathematics, and writing. In addition, adaptive behaviour assessments of functional, habitual everyday skills are useful through interviews with care givers. IQ tests may give some useful information, but a more expanded understanding of cognitive and motor functions in light of the research base on SBM will help elucidate needed interventions. There are few interventions that are specific to people with SBM, although access to the knowledge base is critical. In general, it is important to build on strengths in associative processing, but also focus on generalization across contexts. Interventions that work in other populations (*e.g.* reading and mathematics in learning disabilities) work for those with SBM. Follow standard assessment and intervention procedures, taking into account the differences in how difficulties commonly occur in SBM. Focusing on attention problems is important, but children with SBM do not reliably respond to stimulant medication (Davidovich *et al.*, 1999). Structuring the environment and ensuring consistency of schedules and routines is often very helpful. The brain, and not the spine, leads to attention and learning difficulties. Motivation and laziness rarely account for learning problems in people with SBM, although these factors make them worse.

Schooling can be a very difficult experience for children with SBM because of lack of understanding of the disorder and insufficient appreciation of strengths and weaknesses in academic skills. The strengths (weaknesses) are in reading decoding (not reading comprehension), mathematics facts (not mathematics procedures), vocabulary (not listening comprehension), talking (not writing), and sociability (not attention). Carefully structured academic plans that accommodate weaknesses and also attempt early intervention are especially important.

Psychosocial factors must also be evaluated and treated. In a review of psychosocial and family factors in spina bifida, Holmbeck and colleagues (2006) reported that family dysfunction occurred in about 12 per cent of their sample. Although many families are resilient, parents often report feelings of anxiety and depression related to the burden of care represented by a child with spina bifida. Parents report lack of confidence and worry about the child's future. The child's level of cognitive ability influences parenting because the parents of lower functioning children provide less autonomy and exercise more control. Early intervention addressing parental understanding and parenting that promotes autonomy may be associated with better social and behavioural outcomes. Distressed families should access counselling as early as possible to prevent behavioural patterns between parents and child that are maladaptive.

Conclusions

SBM shows variable outcomes, but the variability is principled. Outcomes are related to physical and neural phenotypes, and likely the genotype. In addition to ambulation and urological difficulties related to level of spinal lesion, major cognitive problems are related to core deficits in timing, attention orienting, and movement. The difficulties are related to the malformations of the cerebellum and corpus callosum, and general effects of hydrocephalus. The modal profile involves strengths in associative processing and weaknesses in assembled processing. Assessments should be comprehensive and interventions should take into account strengths and weaknesses as they occur in the individual person.

Supported by Eunice Kennedy Shriver National Institute of Child Health and Human Development grant *P01 HD35946*. The opinions expressed in this paper are not necessarily the opinions of the NICHD.

Conflicts of interest: none.

References

Au, K.S., Ashley-Koch, A. & Northrup, H. (2010): Epidemiologic and genetic aspects of spina bifida and other neural tube defects. *Dev. Disabil. Res. Rev.* **16**, 6–25.

Barkovich, A.J. & Raybaud, C. (2012): *Pediatric Neuroimaging (5th ed.)*. Philadelphia, PA: Lippincott Williams & Wilkins.

Bowman, R.M. & McLone, D.G. (2010): Neurosurgical management of spina bifida: research issues. *Dev. Disabil. Res. Rev.* **16**, 82–87.

Brewer, V.R., Fletcher, J.M., Hiscock, M. & Davidson, K.C. (2001): Attention processes in children with shunted hydrocephalus versus attention deficit/hyperactivity disorder. *Neuropsychology* **15**, 185–198.

Burmeister, R., Hannay, H.J., Fletcher, J.M., Boudousquie, A. & Dennis, M. (2005): Attention problems and executive functions in children with spina bifida meningomyelocele. *Child Neuropsychol.* **11**, 265–284.

Copp, A.J., Stanier, P. & Greene, N.D.F. (2013): Neural tube defects: recent advances, unsolved questions, and controversies. *Lancet Neurol.* **12**, 799–810.

Davidovitch, M., Manning-Courtney, P., Hartmann, L.A., Watson, J., Lutkenhoff, M. & Oppenheimer, S. (1999): The prevalence of attentional problems and the effect of methylphenidate in children with myelomenigocele. *Pediatr. Rehabil.* **3**, 29–35.

Del Bigio, M.R. (2010): Neuropathology and structural changes in hydrocephalus. *Dev. Disabil. Res. Rev.* **16**, 16–22.

Dennis, M. & Barnes, M. (2010): The cognitive phenotype of spina bifida myelomeningocele. *Dev. Disabil. Res. Rev.* **16**, 31–39.

Dennis, M., Edelstein, K., Copeland, K., *et al.* (2005): Covert orienting to exogenous and endogenous cues in children with spina bifida. *Neuropsychologia* **43**, 976–987.

Dennis, M., Landry, S.H., Barnes, M.H. & Fletcher, J.M. (2006): A model of neurocognitive function in spina bifida over the lifespan: a model of core and functional deficits. *J. Int. Neuropsych. Soc.* **12,** 285–296.

Dennis, M., Sinopoli, K.J., Fletcher, J.M. & Schachar, R. (2008): Puppets, robots, critics, and actors within a taxonomy of attention for developmental disorders. *J. Int. Neuropsych. Soc.* **14,** 673–690.

Dennis, M., Salman, M., Juranek, J. & Fletcher, J.M. (2010): Cerebellar motor function in spina bifida meningomyelocele. *Cerebellum* **9,** 484–498.

Detrait, E.R., George, T.M., Etchevers, H.C., Gilbert, J.R., Vekemans, M. & Speer, M.C. (2005): Human neural tube defects: developmental biology, epidemiology, and genetics. *Neurotoxicol. Teratol.* **27,** 515–524.

Edelstein, K., Dennis, M., Copeland, K., *et al.* (2004): Motor learning in children with spina bifida: dissociation between performance level and acquisition rate. *J. Int. Neuropsych. Soc.* **10,** 877–887.

Fletcher, J.M., Dennis, M., Northrup, H., *et al.* (2004): Spina bifida: genes, brain, and development. In: *International Review of Research in Mental Retardation*, ed. L. Glidden, Vol 29, pp. 63–117. San Diego: Academic Press.

Fletcher, J.M., Copeland, K., Frederick, J., *et al.* (2005): Spinal lesion level in spina bifida meningomyelocele: a source of neural and cognitive heterogeneity. *J. Neurosurg.* **3,** 268–279.

Fletcher, J.M., Ostermaier, K.K., Cirino, P.T. & Dennis, M. (2008): Neurobehavioral outcomes in spina bifida: processes versus outcomes. *J. Ped. Rehab. Med.* **1,** 1–14.

Hannay, H.J., Dennis, M., Kramer, L., Blaser, S. & Fletcher, J.M. (2009): Partial agenesis of the corpus callosum in spina bifida meningomyelocele and potential compensatory mechanisms. *J. Clin. Exp. Neuropsych.* **31,** 180–194.

Hasan, K.M., Eluvathingal, T.J., Kramer, L.A., Ewing-Cobbs, L., Dennis, M. & Fletcher, J.M. (2008a): White matter microstructural abnormalities in children with spina bifida myelomeningocele and hydrocephalus: a diffusion tensor tractography study of the association pathways. *J. Mag. Res. Imag.* **27,** 700–709.

Hasan, K.M., Sankar, A., Halphen, C., *et al.* (2008b): Quantitative diffusion tensor imaging and intellectual outcomes in spina bifida. *J. Neurosurg.* **2,** 75–82.

Herweh, C., Akbar, M., Wengenroth, M., *et al.* (2009): DTI of commissural fibers in patients with Chiari II-malformation. *Neuroimage* **44,** 306–311.

Hetherington, R., Dennis, M., Barnes, M., Drake, J. & Gentili, F. (2006): Functional outcome in young adults with spina bifida and hydrocephalus. *Ch. Nerv. Sys.* **22,** 117–124.

Holmbeck, G.N., Greenley, R.N., Coakley, R.M., Greco, J. & Hagstrom, J. (2006): Family functioning in children and adolescents with spina bifida: an evidence-based review of research and interventions. *Dev. Behav. Ped.* **27,** 249–277.

Juranek, J.J. & Salman, M.S. (2010): Anomalous development of brain structure and function in spina bifida myelomeningocele. *Dev. Disabil. Res. Rev.* **16,** 23–30.

Juranek, J., Fletcher, J.M., Hasan, K.H., *et al.* (2008): Neocortical reorganization in spina bifida. *Neuroimage* **40,** 1516–1522.

Juranek, J.J., Dennis, M., Cirino, P.T., El-Messidi, L. & Fletcher, J.M. (2010): The cerebellum in children with spina bifida and Chiari II malformation: quantitative volumetrics by region. *Cerebellum* **9,** 240–248.

Kulesz, P., Williams, V., Treble-Barna, A., Juranek, J.J., Dennis, M. & Fletcher, J.M. (2014): Quantitative assessment of the tectum and covert orienting in children with spina bifida meningomyelocele. Unpublished manuscript.

Liptak, GS. (2013): Neural tube defects. In: *Children with Disabilities, 7th ed,* eds. M.L. Batshaw, N.J. Roizen, & Lotrecchiano, G.R., pp. 451–472. Baltimore, MD: Paul H. Brookes Publishing.

Ou, X., Glasier, C.M. & Snow, J.H. (2011): Diffusion tensor imaging evaluation of white matter in adolescents with myelomeningocele and Chiari II malformation. *Pediatr. Radiol.* **41,** 1407–1415.

Taylor, H.B., Barnes, M.A., Landry, S.H., Swank, P., Fletcher, J.M. & Huang, F. (2013): Motor contingency learning and infants with spina bifida. *J. Int. Neuropsych. Soc.* **19,** 206–215.

Treble, A., Juranek, J.J., Stuebing, K.K., Dennis, M. & Fletcher, J.M. (2012): Functional significance of atypical cortical organization in spina bifida myelomeningocele: relations of cortical thickness and gyrification with IQ and fine motor dexterity. *Cereb. Cortex* **23,** 2357–2369.

Treble-Barna, A., Juranek, J., Stuebing, K.K., Cirino, P.T., Dennis, M. & Fletcher, J.M. (2015): Prospective and episodic memory in relation to hippocampal volume in adults with spina bifida myelomeningocele. *Neuropsychology* **29**(1), 92-101.

Treble-Barna, A., Kulesz, P., Fletcher, J.M. & Dennis, M. (2014): The effect of posterior fossa dysmorphology on covert orienting: a comparison of three etiologies of congenital hydrocephalus. *J. Int. Neuropsych. Soc.* **20,** 1–10.

Ware, A.L., Juranek, J.J., Williams, V., Cirino, P., Dennis, M. & Fletcher, J.M. (2014): Anatomical and diffusion MRI of deep gray matter in pediatric spina bifida. *Neuroimage Clin.* **5,** 120–127.

Williams, T.J., Juranek, J.J., Stuebing, K.K., Cirino, P.T., Dennis, M. & Fletcher, J.M. (2013): Examination of frontal and parietal tectocortical attention pathways in spina bifida meningomyelocele using probabilistic diffusion tractography. *Brain Connect.* **3,** 512–522.

Chapter 8

Neurocognitive, neuropsychological, and neurovisual development in single-suture craniosynostoses

Daniela Chieffo*° and Luca Massimi°

*Paediatric Neurology and Psychiatry;
°Paediatric Neurosurgery, Catholic University Medical School, A. Gemelli Hospital,
largo A. Gemelli 8, 00168 Rome, Italy
daniela.chieffo@rm.unicatt.it

Summary

Craniosynostoses are characterized by the premature fusion of one or more sutures separating the bony plates of the skull during early development. They can occur as an isolated disorder or be part of a syndrome. Isolated craniosynostosis usually involves one suture (mono-sutural synostosis) and shows a significantly better aesthetic, surgical, and developmental outcome when compared with multi-sutural/syndromic synostosis. However, children affected by mono-sutural synostosis can also have an adverse neurodevelopmental outcome, especially concerning visual, cognitive, language, and motor domains. The goal of this chapter is to present the very latest developments in our understanding of cognitive/neuropsychological and neurovisual aspects regarding sagittal synostosis (SS), unicoronal synostosis (US), and metopic synostosis (MS).

Cognitive and neuropsychological profile

Monosutural non-syndromic craniosynostoses were traditionally thought to be possible causes of impairment of cognitive and neuropsychological functions because of raised intracranial pressure (ICP) and subsequent reduced brain blood inflow, and/or deformation of the brain (Fernbach & Feinstein, 1991; Renier *et al.*, 2000). However, there are several issues that make these topics controversial. Regarding the matter of raised ICP: 1) there are no standardized methods for its measurements, nor values of reference; 2) increased ICP has been demonstrated in a minority of cases (5 to 25 per cent), mainly syndromic or complex synostoses (Bristol *et al.*, 2004; Tamburrini *et al.*, 2005); and 3) the effects of raised ICP on psychomotor development has been specifically investigated with inconclusive results in only a few studies (Arnaud *et al.*, 1995; Gewalli *et al.*, 2001). Similarly, no definite correlation between brain deformation and craniosynostosis has been found so far; brain deformation is expected to be independent of or only partially dependent on synostosis, since it involves not only the superficial areas, but also the deep brain regions and the white matter (Aldridge *et al.*,

2002). Therefore, the current trend is to consider the cognitive and neuropsychological deficits as a consequence of a primary brain dysfunction associated with the craniosynostosis, rather than a brain dysfunction resulting from the craniosynostosis (Kapp-Simon et al., 2007; Starr et al., 2012).

Early outcome

This new understanding is giving rise to an increasing number of neuropsychological studies focusing on children with monosutural synostoses. Accordingly, overall, these children show normal IQ and normal psychomotor development, however, sectorial problems, such as learning or language deficits, can be found in 35 to 40 per cent (3-5 times more than in the normal population), independent of the type of synostosis (Becker et al., 2005; Magge et al., 2002; Shipster et al., 2003; Speltz et al., 2004). However, the matter is relatively complicated and still debated since there is no strict concordance among the different studies, mainly due to the different methods and the different series. Furthermore, as far as the preoperative and the early postoperative period are concerned, some investigations carried out using the Bayley Scales of Infant Development I and II (BSID-I and BSID-II) revealed a Mental Development Index (MDI) and a Psychomotor Development Index (PDI) from moderately to severely worse in 64 per cent and 55 per cent of affected children at diagnosis (SS, MS, US), respectively, compared with normal subjects, without significant changes after surgery (Cohen et al., 2004). Other authors, using BSID only in MS children, found normal MDI scores and a good correlation with maternal instruction, but no correlation with severity of synostosis (Warschausky et al., 2005). In a prospective study of 100 children, Kapp-Simon and coworkers (2005) confirmed the low scores at diagnosis in affected children (MDI: -2/3 SD; PDI: -1 SD), compared to the average (no control subjects were enrolled), without correlation to social and cultural background. An update of the latter study with 125 controls, provided by Speltz and coworkers, showed that even the control population had scores lower than the average (MDI: -1/3 SD; PDI: -0.5 SD) (Speltz et al., 2007), thus raising some doubts about the application of the BSID (Dewey et al., 1998). On the other hand, Bellew and coworkers (2005), using the Griffiths Mental Development Scales (GMDS), tested 28 SS children, 28 healthy controls, and a group of non-surgically treated SS children with the same sociocultural background, and found that SS children presented with a worse score only in the gross motor function scale compared with healthy controls, and that these scores were normalized after surgery. SS children who also received surgery showed a better psychomotor development compared with non-surgically treated subjects (less evident in eye-hand coordination and performance). This data was confirmed over a 5-year follow-up period (Bellew et al., 2011). In summary, according to the extensive and systematic review of the literature recently provided by Knight and colleagues (2014), monosutural synostoses carry an increased preoperative risk of developmental delay in both cognitive and motor domains; particularly for patients belonging to the lower end of the developmental spectrum rather than the higher end when a comparison is made with standard estimates. Cognitive, language, and motor deficits persist early after surgery in most series.

Late outcome

As far as the outcome during childhood and adolescence is concerned, IQ is generally within the average range with appropriate general intellectual functioning at school age, though with a downward shift, with an increased prevalence of language, learning, and behavioural difficulties (Knight *et al.*, 2014). Boltshauer and coworkers found no significant differences regarding IQ scores and neuropsychological deficits (namely in attention, learning, and memory) between 30 SS non-surgically treated children (mean age: 9.25 years) and their healthy siblings (Boltshauser *et al.*, 2003). The different ages between cases and controls and the emotional state of siblings were the main limitations of this study. Da Costa and collaborators (2006) observed normal IQ (both PIQ and VIQ) in subjects with monosutural synostosis, but reduced scores in frontal lobe-related skills (attention, visuo-spatial planning, and problem solving). Similar deficits, but with significantly lower scores, were found in syndromic subjects. In a cohort of adolescents consisting of 35 SS patients (mean age: 13.4 years) and 30 US patients (mean age: 14.9 years), who previously received surgery (mean age at surgery: 7.2 years), we observed selective and sustained attention deficits in 17 per cent SS subjects (7 per cent of whom also showed visuo-spatial and constructional ability defects with associated visual memory recall) and processing and planning speech deficits in 30 per cent of US subjects (Chieffo *et al.*, 2010).

Correlation between suture and specific neurodevelopment

At present, the correlation between type of craniosynostosis or possible related brain damage and psychomotor development is not yet well defined. The theory in which a relationship between involved suture and specific neuropsychological deficit is postulated, indeed, has limitations: 1) the studies addressing specifically the relationship between anatomical damage and corresponding neuropsychological function demonstrated only an increased risk of deficit in the case of cumulative anatomical damage (Leonard *et al.*, 2001); 2) according to high-definition and volumetric neuroimaging investigations, the brain anomalies are not only below the fused suture but also within the white matter, and the volume and shape of the brain is abnormal in both the preoperative and the postoperative period compared with normal subjects, thus reinforcing the idea of a primary brain dysfunction (Aldridge *et al.*, 2005a, 2005b, 2002; Paniagua *et al.*, 2013); 3) monosutural craniosynostoses are thought to have a multifactorial aetiology; therefore, the related neuropsychological deficits could also have the same genesis; Moreover, 4) neuropsychological functions would be little affected by the synostosis because of the influence of neuronal plasticity, socio-cultural background, adaptation skills, and so on. In spite of these limitations, however, a neuropsychological profile for each type of synostosis has been traced:

a) Sagittal synostosis (the most widely investigated). SS children usually present with early language development disorders with later learning, working memory, attention, and planning defects, similar to what is observed for attention deficit/hyperactivity disturbance (ADHD) (Kapp-Simon *et al.*, 2007). The anatomical background may relate to the bilateral deformation of the sylvian and parieto-occipital regions, and the dorso-lateral areas of the prefrontal cortex. A recent study based on 3T MRI of SS children showed impaired brain connectivity, correlating with the aforementioned neuropsychological deficits, in particular, concerning the pathways afferent to the prefrontal cortex, the anterior and posterior cingulate cortex, the precuneus, the parahyppocampus, and the left angular gyrus (Beckett *et al.*, 2014).

b) Metopic synostosis. Based on the poor information available to date, MS children mainly show learning and behavioural problems (Becker *et al.*, 2005; Demer, 2006). The bilateral distortion of the frontal lobe (reduced volume?) would explain the cognitive retardation in some subjects (Bottero *et al.*, 1998).

6) Little can be said about the factors influencing neurodevelopmental outcome. According to the aforementioned systematic literature review (Knight *et al.*, 2014) no statistically significant data about intrinsic factors can be obtained by analyzing brain imaging (the study on brain connectivity by Beckett and colleagues was not included since it was not yet published), the degree of skull deformity, the type of synostosis, genetics, or gender. Similar considerations can be made for extrinsic factors, such as maternal intelligence or education, and the socio-economic background. The early age at surgery (within the first year of life) was associated with a better outcome in earlier studies, whereas such a correlation was not confirmed in recent, methodologically more rigorous studies. Finally, the age at evaluation was shown to have a direct correlation with speech-language and cognitive deficits (the older the age at evaluation, the higher the percentage of deficits) in the series of Becker and collaborators (2005) (SS, US, and MS patients) and in the series of Mendonca and colleagues (2009) (only MS subjects).

Neurovisual functions

Most of the studies concerning the visual functions in craniosynostoses are focused on the ocular and orbital abnormalities in syndromic patients and their consequences. About 50-70 per cent of these children are actually affected by visual deficits (namely, strabismus, astigmatism, and acuity defects) as a result of orbital distortion, proptosis, and keratosis (Khan *et al.*, 2003; Tay *et al.*, 2006). On the other hand, only a few studies have addressed monosutural synostoses, mainly due to a low expected incidence of visual problems and, in particular, the complexity to test small infants in the preoperative period. Therefore, most of the data available results form series in which children with monosutural synostoses are mixed with syndromic children (and often monosutural synostosis is part of the syndrome) or from series consisting of non-surgically treated children or children tested in the late postoperative period. Accordingly, US children are burdened by (vertical) strabismus resulting from the flattening of the orbit and the deformation of the anterior skull base, with later impaired growth of the intraorbital muscles and tendons (Bagolini *et al.*, 1982; Limon de Brown *et al.*, 1988). Similarly, the small-sized orbits and the hypotelorism proper of MS may cause compression on the ocular bulb, the trochlea, and the extrinsic ocular muscles with later impairment of ocular movements (Denis *et al.*, 1996).

New methods for assessment

In the last two decades, the feasibility to test children of less than 1 year old has significantly increased with the development of specific examination techniques that allow some visual responses, such as fixation or following, to be elicited, even in preterm neonates (Dubowitz *et al.*, 1983). These so-called behaviour and neuropsychological techniques currently provide the opportunity to reliably assess visual acuity, the visual field, colour discrimination or ocular movements in craniosynostotic infants. A study using these techniques to investigate the main visual functions in the preoperative period (ocular movements, fixation, following, visual acuity, visual field, and visual attention) indicated some interesting and unexpected results (Ricci *et al.*, 2007). The percentage of subjects with normal scores in all tests was actually as low as 15 per cent; 20 per cent had acuity defects and the remaining deficits varied according to the different synostosis. Indeed, children with US showed ocular movements and visual field defects in more than 50 per cent of cases, possibly due to orbital flattening and lateral deviation of the head, as demonstrated by other authors in older subjects (Gupta *et al.*, 2003), as well as those with MS showing ocular movement imbalance in 67 per cent of cases. Surprisingly, about

70 per cent of children with SS had a visual deficit, mainly concerning visual attention (measured by the fixation shift test), which, for a synostosis that does not involve the orbits, can be considered as a "dysfunction" of the parietal lobes (Mercuri et al., 1996).

Early and late outcome: personal experience

Analysis of early postoperative and long-term outcome, according to the personal experience of the aforementioned 48 children (unpublished data), in whom the visual functions were tested preoperatively, 2, 6 and 12 months after surgery and at school age (for methods, refer to Ricci et al. [2007] and Vasco et al. [2008]), showed the following results. In the preoperative period, there were no substantial differences among the different synostoses as far as refractive (18 cases; 37.5 per cent) and acuity deficits were concerned (8 cases; 16.5 per cent). No significant differences were found in visual field defects, even though US patients were predominant (45 per cent *versus* 25 per cent MS and 12 per cent SS), or in the fixation shift test, where SS children were prevalent (48 per cent *versus* 33 per cent MS and 18 per cent US). On the other hand, a statistically significant difference was found among children with strabismus, of whom six of eight were affected by US, and in the fixation and following test which revealed abnormal results in 67 per cent MS and 55 per cent US children, but only in 12 per cent SS children. Within the first year after surgery, no changes in refractive or ocular movement deficits were observed, while the visual acuity, fixation, and follow test, as well as the fixation shift test, became normalized in all cases, except one child with SS. At school age, strabismus persisted in six children; contrast, stereopsis, and crowding tests were normal in all cases. Motor coordination was impaired in three SS children (6.2 per cent) and borderline in six patients (12.5 per cent; three with US and three with MS); in these cases, the body coordination, and both static and dynamic balance were deficient, while the fine coordination was normal. Visuo-perceptual functions were impaired in six cases (12.5 per cent; four SS and two US children), while the perception of movement was borderline in 10 cases (21 per cent; all SS children).

Conclusions

These studies, which are the only currently available for this topic, provide the following main points of discussion.

1) As demonstrated in older children with syndromic synostosis, infants with monosutural synostosis also have a high incidence of visual deficits at diagnosis (80 per cent). Refractive deficits, which are not affected by the synostosis, do not change after surgery and show the same evolution compared to the normal population. On the contrary, all the other deficits quickly improve after surgery to normalization (80 per cent of affected patients normalized within the first year after surgery, 96 per cent within school age), except for ocular movement defects. Such an improvement effectively differentiates monosutural from syndromic synostoses.

2) The detected visual deficits appear to be craniosynostosis-specific. The cranial and, in particular, orbital decompression, which favours normal development of the orbital content (ocular bulb, muscles, tendons, vascular, and neural structures) may account for the significant postoperative improvement of visual acuity, visual field, and fixation and following abilities in affected children (namely, US and MS patients). Similarly, the bi-parietal decompression in SS patients would explain the normalization of the fixation shift in these subjects. The latter

improvement would result from the removal of the mechanical effects of the bi-parietal narrowing rather than the relief from raised intracranial pressure that, in turn, was not clinically demonstrated in the preoperative period.

3) A spontaneous improvement of visual functions should be excluded based on the very rapid response after surgery (already appreciable at two months of follow-up) and the absence of correlation between the clinical improvement and the patient's age at diagnosis, surgery, and follow-up.

4) Strabismus persists in most of the affected children even at late follow-up. As mentioned, strabismus was a burden for almost exclusively US children, for whom the lack of postoperative improvement may have been due to the persistence of a certain lateral deviation of the head, up to the second/third year of age (as found in three of our patients) and/or a suboptimal decompression of the orbit (Demer, 2006). This second hypothesis is supported by the evidence that the patients with more severe forms of US (namely, type IIa, IIb and III) maintain a certain degree of orbital deformation up to adulthood, due to the abnormal development of the skull base (Pelo et al., 2011).

5) About 1 in 10 children (12.5 per cent) show some vision-related cognitive deficits at late follow-up. The most relevant deficits concern motor coordination, especially static and dynamic balance and ability to perform ball exercises (where the position of the body has to be continuously adapted to a moving object and where the ball has to be thrown to a defined place). On these grounds, one could speculate on the negative influence of the preoperative visual deficits on the development of the brain associative areas devoted to the organization of body movement, in spite of normal, final visual development. Such a theory would be confirmed by the low scores of the affected patients based on the Atkinson tests, in which the visuo-perceptual skills are assessed; vision is not sufficient to decode the information since affected children are not able to correctly reproduce the 3D figures by only looking at them; they need to see how they are designed or be able to touch them.

Conflicts of interest: none.

References

Aldridge, K., Kane, A.A., Marsh, J.L., et al. (2005): Brain morphology in nonsyndromic unicoronal craniosynostosis. *Anat. Rec. A. Discov. Mol. Cell. Evol. Biol.* **285,** 690–698.

Aldridge, K., Kane, A.A., Marsh, J.L., Yan, P., Govier, D. & Richtsmeier, J.T. (2005): Relationship of brain and skull in pre- and postoperative sagittal synostosis. *J. Anat.* **206,** 373–38.

Aldridge, K., Marsh, J.L., Govier, D. & Richtsmeier, J.T. (2002): Central nervous system phenotypes in craniosynostosis. *J. Anat.* **201,** 31–39.

Arnaud, E., Renier, D. & Marchac, D. (1995): Prognosis for mental function in scaphocephaly. *J. Neurosurg.* **83,** 476–479.

Bagolini, B., Campos, E.C. & Chiesi, C. (1982): Plagiocephaly causing superior oblique deficiency and ocular torticollis. A new clinical entity. *Arch. Ophthalmol.* **100,** 1093–1096.

Becker, D.B., Petersen, J.D., Kane, A.A., Cradock, M.M., Pilgram, T.K. & Marsh, J.L. (2005): Speech, cognitive, and behavioural outcomes in nonsyndromic craniosynostosis. *Plast. Reconstr. Surg.* **116,** 400–407.

Beckett, J.S., Brooks, E.D., Lacadie, C., et al. (2014): Altered brain connectivity in sagittal craniosynostosis. *J. Neurosurg. Pediatr.* **13,** 690–698.

Bellew, M., Chumas, P.D., Mueller, R., Liddington, M. & Russell, J. (2005): Pre- and postoperative developmental attainment in sagittal synostosis. *Arch. Dis. Child* **90,** 346–350.

Bellew, M., Liddington, M., Chumas, P. & Russell, J. (2011): Preoperative and postoperative developmental attainment in patients with sagittal synostosis: 5-year follow-up. *J. Neurosurg. Pediatr.* **7,** 121–126.

Boltshauser, E., Ludwig, S., Dietrich, F. & Landolt, M.A. (2003): Sagittal craniosynostosis: cognitive, development, behavior, and quality of life in unoperated children. *Neuropediatrics* **34,** 293–300.

Bottero, L., Lajeunie, E., Arnaud, E., Marchac, D. & Renier, D. (1998): Functional outcome after surgery for trigonocephaly. *Plast. Reconstr. Surg.* **102,** 952–958.

Bristol, R.E., Lekovic, G.P. & Rekate, H.L. (2004): The effects of craniosynostosis on the brain with respect to intracranial pressure. *Semin. Pediatr. Neurol.* **11,** 262–267.

Chieffo, D., Tamburrini, G., Massimi, L., et al. (2010): Long-term neuropsychological development in single-suture craniosynostosis treated early. *J. Neurosurg. Pediatr.* **5,** 232–237.

Cohen, S.R., Cho, D.C., Nichols, S.L., Simms, C., Cross, K.P. & Burstein, F.D. (2004): American Society of Maxillofacial Surgeons Outcome Study: preoperative and postoperative neurodevelopmental findings in single-suture craniosynostosis. *Plast. Reconstr. Surg.* **114,** 841–847.

Da Costa, A.C., Anderson, V.A., Savarirayan, R., et al. (2012): Neurodevelopmental functioning of infants with untreated single-suture craniosynostosis during early infancy. *Childs Nerv. Syst.* **28,** 869–877.

Da Costa, A.C., Walters, I., Savarirayan, R., Anderson, V.A., Wrennall, J. & Meara, J.G. (2006): Intellectual outcomes in children and adolescents with syndromic and nonsyndraomic craniosynostosis. *Plast. Reconstr. Surg.* **118,** 175–181.

Demer, J.L. (2006): Current concepts of mechanical and neural factors in ocular motility. *Curr. Opin. Neurol.* **9,** 4–13.

Denis, D., Genitori, L., Conrath, J., Lena, G. & Choux, M. (1996): Ocular findings in children operated on for plagiocephaly and trigonocephaly. *Childs Nerv. Syst.* **12,** 683–689.

Dewey, C., Fleming, P. & Golding, J. (1998): Does the supine sleeping position have any adverse effects on the child? II. Development in the first 18 months. ALSPAC Study Team. *Pediatrics* **101,** E5.

Dubowitz, L.M., Mushin, J., Morante, A. & Placzek, M. (1983): The maturation of visual acuity in neurologically normal and abnormal newborn infants. *Behav. Brain Res.* **10,** 39–45.

Fernbach, S.K. & Feinstein, K.A. (1991): Radiologic evaluation of children with craniosynostosis. *Neurosurg. Clin. N. Am.* **2,** 569–586.

Gewalli, F., Guimaraes-Ferreira, J.P., Sahlin, P., et al. (2001): Mental development after modified pi procedure: dynamic cranioplasty for sagittal synostosis. *Ann. PLast. Surg.* **46,** 415–420.

Greenberg, B.M. & Schneider, S.J. (2006): Trigonocephaly: surgical considerations and long term evaluation. *J. Craniofac. Surg.* **17,** 528–535.

Gupta, P.C., Foster, J., Crowe, S., Papay, F.A., Luciano, M. & Traboulsi, E.I. (2003): Ophthalmologic findings in patients with nonsyndromic plagiocephaly. *J. Craniofac. Surg.* **14,** 529–532.

Hunter, A.G. & Rudd, N.L. (1977): Coronal synostosis: its familial characteristics and associated clinical findings in 109 patients lacking bilateral polysyndactyly or syndactyly. *Teratology* **15,** 301–310.

Kapp-Simon, K.A., Collett, B.R., Barr-Schinzel, M.A., et al. (2012): Behavioral adjustment of toddler and preschool-aged children with single-suture craniosynostosis. *Plast. Reconstr. Surg.* **130,** 635–647.

Kapp-Simon, K.A., Leroux, B., Cunningham, M.L. & Speltz, M.L. (2005): Multi-site study of infants with single-suture craniosynostosis: preliminary report of pre-surgery development. *Cleft Palate Craniofac. J.* **42,** 377–384.

Kapp-Simon, K.A., Speltz, M.L., Cunningham, M.L., Patel, P.K. & Tomita, T. (2007): Neurodevelopment of children with single-suture craniosynostosis: a review. *Childs Nerv. Syst.* **23,** 269–28.

Khan, S.H., Nischal, K.K., Dean, F., Hayward, R.D. & Walker, J. (2003): Visual outcomes and amblyogenic risk factors in craniosynostotic syndromes: a review of 141 cases. *Br. J. Ophthalmol.* **87,** 999–1003.

Knight, S.J., Anderson, V.A., Spencer-Smith, M.M. & Da Costa, A.C. (2014): Neurodevelopmental outcomes in infants and children with single-suture craniosynostosis: a systematic review. *Dev. Neuropsychol.* **39,** 159–186.

Leonard, C.M., Eckert, M.A., Lombardino, L.J., et al. (2001): Anatomical risk factors for phonological dyslexia. *Cereb. Cortex* **11,** 148–157.

Limon de Brown, E., Ortiz Monasterio, F. & Stark Feldman, M. (1988): Strabismus in plagiocephaly. *J. Pediatr. Ophthalmol. Strabismus* **25,** 180–190.

Magge, S.N., Westerveld, M., Pruzinsky, T. & Persing, J.A. (2002): Long-term neuropsychological effects of sagittal craniosynostosis on child development. *J. Craniofac. Surg.* **13,** 99–104.

Mendonca, D.A., White, N., West, E., Dover, S., Solanki, G. & Nishikawa, H. (2009): Is there a relationship between the severity of metopic synostosis and speech and language impairments? *J. Craniofac. Surg.* **20,** 85–88.

Mercuri, E., Atkinson, J., Braddick, O., et al. (1996): Visual function and perinatal focal cerebral infarction. *Arch. Dis. Child.* **75,** F76–F81.

Paniagua, B., Emodi, O., Hill, J., et al. (2013): 3D of brain shape and volume after cranial vault remodeling surgery for craniosynostosis correction in infants. *Proc. Soc. Photo. Opt. Instrum. Eng.* **29**, 8672: 86720V.

Pelo, S., Tamburrini, G., Marianetti, T.M., et al. (2011): Correlations between the abnormal development of the skull base and facial skeleton growth in anterior synostotic plagiocephaly: the predictive value of a classification based on CT scan classification. *Childs Nerv. Syst.* **27**, 1431–1443.

Renier, D., Lajeunie, E., Arnaud, E. & Marchac, D. (2000): Management of craniosynostosis. *Childs Nerv. Syst.* **16**, 645–658.

Ricci, D., Vasco, G., Baranello, G., et al. (2007): Visual function in infants with non-syndromic craniosynostosis. *Dev. Med. Child Neurol.* **49**, 574–576.

Shipster, C., Hearst, D., Somerville, A., Stackhouse, J., Hayward, R. & Wade, A. (2003): Speech, language, and cognitive development in children with isolated sagittal synostosis. *Dev. Med. Child. Neurol.* **45**, 34–43.

Speltz, M.L., Kapp-Simon, K.A., Collett, B., et al. (2007): Neurodevelopment of infants with single-suture craniosynostosis: pre-surgery comparisons with case-matched controls. *Plast. Reconstr. Surg.* **119**, 1874–1881.

Speltz, M.L., Kapp-Simon, K.A., Cunningham, M., Marsh, J. & Dawson, G. (2004): Single-suture craniosynostosis: a review of neurobehavioral research and theory. *J. Pediatr. Psychol.* **29**, 651–668.

Starr, J.R., Collett, B.R., Gaither, R., et al. (2012): Multicenter study of neurodevelopment in 3-year-old children with and without single-suture craniosynostosis. *Arch. Pediatr. Adolesc. Med.* **166**, 536–542.

Tamburrini, G., Caldarelli, M., Massimi, L., Santini, P. & Di Rocco, C. (2005): Intracranial pressure monitoring in children with single suture and complex craniosynostosis: a review. *Childs Nerv. Syst.* **21**, 913–921.

Tay, T., Martin, F., Rowe, N., et al. (2006): Prevalence and causes of visual impairment in craniosynostotic syndromes. *Clin. Experiment Ophthalmol.* **34**, 434–440.

Vasco, G., Baranello, G., Ricci, D., et al. (2008): Longitudinal assessment of visual development in non-syndromic craniosynostosis: a 1-year pre- and post-surgical study. *Arch. Dis. Child.* **93**, 932–935.

Warschausky, S., Angobaldo, J., Kewman, D., Buchman, S., Muraszko, K.M. & Azengart, A. (2005): Early development of infants with untreated metopic craniosynostosis. *Plast. Reconstr. Surg.* **115**, 1518–1523.

Chapter 9

Cognitive and behavioural outcome in children with posterior fossa malformations

Sara Bulgheroni, Fabiana Cazzaniga, Michela Bonalumi and Daria Riva

*Developmental Neurology Division, Fondazione IRCCS Istituto Neurologico 'C. Besta',
via Celoria 11, 20133 Milan, Italy*
bulgheroni.s@istituto-besta.it

Summary

Posterior fossa brain malformations principally involve the cerebellum and cause neuropsychological deficits and/or neurodevelopmental disorders, in particular, intellectual disability, severe language impairments, and emotional-behavioural problems of varying entities, including, at times, autistic-like features. The importance of early diagnosis and treatment implicates the need to monitor the clinical and neuropsychological progression of patients in an attempt to define the impact of these malformations on their long-term neurodevelopmental outcome. The purpose underlying these efforts is to learn how to manage these patients in such a way as to promote a better quality of life and a more favourable adaptation to their environment. This chapter will attempt to provide a review of the studies outlined in the literature concerning some profiles of posterior fossa brain malformations, and data from our own archives are presented whenever possible. Until now, a large number of articles on this topic suggests that children with isolated inferior vermian hypoplasia and mega cisterna magna tend to have a positive outcome, while those with vermian hypoplasia and cerebellar agenesis malformations appear to show a moderate or severe degree of neurodevelopmental delay. Although results concerning the Dandy-Walker malformation (DWM) are not entirely conclusive, they consistently suggest that the presence of a well-lobulated cerebellar vermis and the absence of associated brain abnormalities are correlated to a better cognitive outcome. Joubert syndrome (JS), featured by the neuroimaging finding of a molar tooth, appears to have a more heterogeneous outcome, characterized in the majority of patients by slight-to-moderate intellectual disability, frequently accompanied by severely compromised expressive language, good conservation of non-verbal communication modalities, and relatively conserved emotional-behavioural functioning. The preliminary results of the Italian Joubert Syndrome Study Group will also be outlined.

Introduction

Recent advances in neonatal intensive care and neuroimaging techniques, in particular magnetic resonance imaging (MRI), have greatly improved our ability to detect structural anomalies in the posterior fossa. The incidence of posterior fossa malformations diagnosed in the newborn period is estimated to be 1 in every 5,000 live births (Bolduc & Limperopoulos, 2009). Although the exact prevalence in unknown, posterior fossa malformations evaluated by foetal MRI are now among the most common brain malformations detected development, expressive language, as well as gross and fine motor skills. As expected, decreased volume in the right lateral cerebellar hemisphere was related to impaired cognition, in particular, expressive language, and also to gross motor function. Additionally, reduced vermis volume was associated with impaired global development, expressive language, and gross and fine motor skills, as well as behavioural problems and a higher rate of positive autism spectrum scores. These results, which have begun to define the structural topography of functional outcome in children with CBMs, could lead to greater accuracy of prognostication.

Besides the studies considering subjects with CBM as a single sample, there is a growing body of literature in which specific diagnostic and MRI subgroups are being investigated. The posterior fossa malformations usually present a neuroimaging pattern characterized by cerebellar hypoplasia with mainly vermis involvement (Poretti *et al.*, 2014).

The most striking of these anomalies is the DWM, in which an enlarged cerebrospinal fluid (CSF) space results from cystic dilation of the fourth ventricle with complete or partial agenesis of the cerebellar vermis, hypoplasia of the cerebellar hemispheres, and enlargement of the posterior fossa combined with elevation of the torcula and anterior displacement of the brainstem; some authors include other features such as the presence of hydrocephalus (Limperopoulos & du Plessis, 2006). The DWM, Dandy-Walker variant (DWV) without enlargement of the posterior fossa, and MCM are classified as a continuum of developmental anomalies, termed the "Dandy-Walker complex" (DWC).

There are inconsistencies in the outcomes of DWM patients. Up to one third of all patients are reported to develop normally (Ecker *et al.*, 2000; Klein *et al.*, 2003; Kölble *et al.*, 2000; Sasaki-Adams *et al.*, 2008). Intellectual disability appears to be more frequent in DWM cases in which there is abnormal vermis lobulation (Klein *et al.*, 2003; Boddaert *et al.*, 2003) and associated supratentorial abnormalities (Boddaert *et al.*, 2003), such as ventriculomegaly and agenesis of the corpus callosum. Language and communication abilities have not been extensively described. In 2013, Graf and colleagues suggested to consider CCAS symptoms as an integral feature of the DWC and presented the case of a 26-year-old DWV patient who showed low-average intelligence quotient, attention deficits, impulse-control problems, below-average performance in visual short-term memory, verbal and working memory, and general impairments in executive functioning, such as planning and problem solving.

MCM is characterized by an enlarged cisterna magna with a normal fourth ventricle and cerebellar hemispheres and vermis. The developmental outcome of children with MCM has generally been described as favourable, and the majority of those (92 to 100 per cent) with the isolated form appear to develop normally (Forzano *et al.*, 2007; Long *et al.*, 2006; Haimovici *et al.*, 1997). Twenty-nine children with enlargement of the cisterna magna identified *in utero* were compared to 35 children whose foetal ultrasound had been normal (Dror *et al.*, 2009). The two samples had overall performance within the normal range; their mean performance was practically equivalent if the four subjects with borderline developmental quotient were excluded from the MCM group. There were no differences in motor performance between the two samples although walking age was significantly delayed in the MCM group (mean age: approximately 15 months). A study of 18 adults with isolated MCM found that the patients had normal intelligence but that their performance on the memory tasks and verbal and semantic fluency was slightly inferior to that of controls (Zimmer *et al.*, 2007). It can be postulated that more subtle deficits went undetected because sensitive neuropsychological testing was not employed in the reviewed paediatric studies; it is also possible that some higher cognitive deficits present only later in life.

Isolated inferior vermina hypoplasia (iiVH) with normal cerebellar hemispheres and brainstem is an inconsistently used diagnostic entity. Some authors consider iiVH a normal variant, while others refer to it as a DWV variant despite the fact that it lacks a cystic fourth ventricle and has a normal-size posterior fossa. The risk of over-diagnosing the lesion was emphasized by Limperopoulos and colleagues (2006), who showed that 32 per cent (6 of 19) of iiVH cases diagnosed by foetal MRI in the second trimester were normal on postnatal MRI. The study raised important questions about the sensitivity and specificity of foetal MRI and about possible normal variations in the time course of vermian development. More recent studies suggest that subjects diagnosed with iiVH have a rather favourable prognosis. Limperopoulos and collaborators (2006) compared prenatal and postnatal MRI studies in subjects diagnosed with iiVH; the disorder was confirmed in 13 of the 19 patients. The results of this study also indicated that mean gross and fine motor, expressive language, and developmental performance scores were significantly higher in the infants with normal postnatal MRI, compared to those with confirmed postnatal iiVH. Similarly, mean scores in the communication, socialization, and motor domains of the Vineland Adaptive Behaviour Scale were significantly lower among the infants with confirmed diagnosis, compared to those with normal postnatal MRI. Emotional functioning and behaviour were characterized by internalizing problems. Indeed, a subject-by-subject analysis found that only 3 of 13 confirmed cases showed significant neurodevelopmental delay and two had internalizing behaviour problems; the prognosis was thus generally favourable.

The findings of Tarui and collaborators (2014) confirmed an adequate long-term neurodevelopmental outcome in 20 school-aged iiVH children. A subgroup of children (2/20) demonstrating cognitive delay and behavioural impairments had more extensive cerebellar malformation. Finally, as a postnatal confirmed diagnosis of iiVH is associated with persistent elevated parental stress, despite normal developmental outcomes, counselling and ongoing support appear to be indicated in these cases.

As the development of the cerebellum and brainstem are intimately connected, it is not surprising that malformation of the cerebellum and brainstem often occur together. JS is a typical example of these conditions. It is one of the most common inherited congenital ataxias, characterized by a peculiar mid-hindbrain malformation known as the "molar tooth sign" (MTS). This complex defect is characterized by variable degrees of cerebellar vermian hypodysplasia associated with a deepened interpeduncular fossa and thickened, elongated, and mal-oriented superior cerebellar peduncles, giving the overall appearance of a "molar tooth" on axial brain MRI sections (Maria *et al.*, 1997). The absence of decussation of the superior cerebellar peduncles, as well as the cortical spinal tract at the medullary pyramids, are other typical findings (Poretti *et al.*, 2007).

JS is characterized by marked clinical and genetic heterogeneity. The neurological presentation of the disorder includes hypotonia, ataxia, developmental delay often associated with intellectual disability, altered respiratory pattern during the neonatal period, abnormal ocular movements, and distinctive facial features. These neurological signs can be associated with variable multi-organ involvement, mainly of the retina, kidneys, liver, and skeleton.

Twenty-seven causative genes with autosomal or X-linked recessive inheritance have been identified until now. Interestingly, all genes were found to encode for proteins of the primary cilium, making JS part of the expanding family of ciliopathies, a group of heterogeneous conditions sharing both clinical features and genetic determinants (Romani *et al.*, 2013; Beck *et al.*, 2014).

Cognitive and affective development in a few children diagnosed with JS has been investigated in recent years in an effort to define the cognitive and behavioural phenotype of this syndrome. Most studies have confirmed that developmental delay and mild-to-severe intellectual disability are key features of JS; in exceptional cases, patients may have borderline (Steinlin et al., 1997; Fennell et al., 1999; Tavano & Borgatti, 2010) or even normal intelligence (Poretti et al., 2009; Gunay-Aygun et al., 2009; Romani et al., 2013). The finding of siblings discordant for cognitive development has further confirmed the difficulty in predicting the long-term outcome (Steinlin et al., 1997; Poretti et al., 2009).

Based on the first long-term study of 19 JS children, Steinlin and colleagues (1997) divided the outcome of the syndrome into three possible courses: three children died before the age of three, nine had a mildly delayed developmental quotient (DQ) ranging from 60 to 85, and four had a DQ of 30 or less and severe visual and motor problems.

Fennell and collaborators (1999) described a variety of cognitive, verbal memory, visuomotor, fine motor control, and language-related task deficits in 10 of 40 assessable children. Deficits in cognition, verbal fluency and memory, and picture recognition vocabulary were, in particular, identified by standardised tests, however, the sample size was relatively small, i.e. two to four children. Parental reports, moreover, showed that only three of the 40 children were within the borderline range, with the rest scoring in the severely impaired range.

In addition to intellectual disability, language deficit is also considered a constant feature of JS, ranging from complete absence of language, with or without use of gestures, to more understandable speech with severe-to-moderate impairment in both the expressive and receptive domains.

Ozonoff and colleagues (1999) reported that only four of the 11 children with JS studied were verbal and only three of 10 used adequate non-verbal behaviour to regulate social interaction. These results suggest that autism spectrum disorders and associated communication impairments might be common in JS, as confirmed by Hodgkins and collaborators (2004) who described common communicative deficit and autistic-like behaviours (severe temper tantrums that appeared to correlate with difficulty in verbal production) in a group of 29 JS patients.

Reporting on 21 individuals (between 32 months and 19 years of age) with a diagnosis of JS, Braddock and colleagues (2006) described a distinct oro-motor pattern consistent with verbal and lingual apraxias, despite effective gesture production particularly in those whose speech was less intelligible; these results are consistent with those of another study indicating that persons with JS typically do not exhibit classic symptoms of autism spectrum disorder (Takahashi et al., 2005).

More recently, Tavano and Borgatti (2010) compared the neurobehavioural profiles of JS children with those who had malformations confined to the cerebellar vermis and one or both hemispheres. Their findings support the hypothesis that cerebellar structures play an important role in shaping emotional, cognitive, and linguistic development when vermian lesions are associated with cerebellar hemispheric lesions. Cerebellar vermis and brainstem lesions, instead, appear to have a major impact on motor-related skills, including oro-motor abilities and verbal working memory.

The Italian Joubert Syndrome Study Group recently set out to carry out a prospective evaluation of a large sample of JS patients using comprehensive and standardized neuropsychological and behavioural instruments. Fifty-four patients (35 males, 19 females; age range: 10 months to 29 years; median age: 8 years and 5 months; mean age: 9 years and 11months; SD: 6 years and 6 months) were selected between 2007 and 2010 by the Italian Scientific Institutes and

Universities specialized in the management of JS subjects. All patients had MRI showing evidence of MTS. Each underwent a neurological evaluation as well as psychiatric, neuropsychological, and neurolinguistic assessment using standardized norm-referenced, age-appropriate instruments to assess intelligence, language, and adaptive and affective behaviour (more details on the neuropsychological protocol are available in Bulgheroni et al., 2014). Intellectual functioning was found to be remarkably variable with full IQ scores ranging between 32 and 129. Five subjects were not assessable using standardized instruments. Sixteen had IQs within the normal range; about half of these had preserved non-verbal intellectual abilities in the presence of unintelligible speech due to severe dysarthria, according to the Leiter-R, a standardized non-verbal intelligence test that can be used for a number of different population types.

It is known that expressive language skills are generally more affected than either lexical or morpho-syntactic comprehension, a pattern that may be influenced by a concomitant presence of speech dyspraxia. Our data on a subset of 20 of these patients confirmed that the lexical and morpho-syntactic comprehension resulted comparable or superior to the patients' lexical competence based on picture naming. Language abilities were adequate for the patients' general cognitive development, however, it should be noticed that seven subjects from the total sample were pre-verbal.

With regards to adaptive behaviour, the Vineland Adaptive Behaviour Scale quotient was not found to be lower than the intelligence quotient. Verbal abilities in everyday life were relatively preserved, with higher scores in the communication domain, relative to both the daily living and socialization quotients. The test confirmed that the motor domain is the area of greatest vulnerability in JS with a negative impact on many aspects of adaptive behaviour by limiting the acquisition of personal care abilities (dressing and personal hygiene), social interaction (group play and sport skills), and school-related skills (drawing and writing).

Most children did not show maladaptive behaviours that could be considered consistent with a psychiatric diagnosis, but a subset of approximately 40 per cent displayed significant problems in areas such as inattention, overactivity, social withdrawal, and atypical behaviours.

In summary, development of children with JS is characterized by relatively preserved behavioural functioning but impairment in expressive language and short-term memory. Approximately 30 per cent of the patients studied had borderline to normal cognition.

Conclusions

Posterior fossa malformations are usually associated with neuropsychological impairments and\or various neurodevelopmental disorders such as intellectual disabilities, language disorders, and behavioural changes to the autistic phenotype (Riva et al., 2000; Tavano et al., 2007a; Bolduc et al., 2011a). The phenotypes range from mild clinical impairment, even when cerebellar agenesis is nearly complete (Tavano et al., 2007b), to serious neurological, developmental, and functional disabilities (Bolduc et al., 2011b). The clinical picture is generally more serious when the cerebellar vermis is damaged, although exceptions have been noted, as in the case of DWM and iiVH; the presence of supratentorial abnormalities and chromosomal alterations are predictors of poor outcome.

Advances in pre- and neonatal MRI have made it possible to detect increasingly smaller and more subtle cerebellar structural abnormalities. Since the detection of posterior fossa abnormalities in utero has been associated with a termination rate of up to 80 per cent (Adamsbaum et al., 2005), rigorous outcome studies are urgently needed to delineate the long-term clinical significance of small subtle abnormalities that are now being detected. The findings produced will help to guide clinicians as they counsel and support parents with a foetus in whom a posterior fossa anomaly is suspected.

A multidisciplinary approach should be used to study the neuropsychological and neurobehavioural features of large cohorts of patients with posterior fossa malformations selected following rigorous neurological and neuroimaging criteria, in an attempt to collect and analyze longitudinal data on this population.

Conflicts of interest: none.

References

Adamsbaum, C., Moutard, M.L., André, C., et al. (2005): MRI of the fetal posterior fossa. *Pediatr. Radiol.* **35,** 124–140.

Attig, E., Botez, M.I., Hublet, C., Vervonck, C., Jacquy, J. & Capon, A. (1991): Cerebral crossed diaschisis caused by cerebellar lesion: role of the cerebellum in mental functions. *Rev. Neurol. (Paris)* **147,** 200–207.

Baillieux, H., De Smet, H.J., Dobbeleir, A., Paquier, P.F., De Deyn, P.P. & Mariën, P. (2010): Cognitive and affective disturbances following focal cerebellar damage in adults: a neuropsychological and SPECT study. *Cortex* **46,** 869–879.

Beck, B.B., Philipps, J.B., Bartram, M.P., et al. (2014): Mutation of POC1B in a severe syndromic retinal ciliopathy. *Hum. Mutat.* **35,** 1153-1162.

Boddaert, N., Klein, O., Ferguson, N., et al. (2003): Intellectual prognosis of the Dandy-Walker malformation in children: the importance of vermian lobulation. *Neuroradiology* **45,** 320–324.

Bolduc, M.E. & Limperopoulos, C. (2009): Neurodevelopmental outcomes in children with cerebellar malformations: a systematic review. *Dev. Med. Child Neurol.* **51,** 256–267.

Bolduc, M.E., Du Plessis, A.J., Sullivan, N., et al. (2011a): Spectrum of neurodevelopmental disabilities in children with cerebellar malformations. *Dev. Med. Child Neurol.* **53,** 409–416.

Bolduc, M.E., Du Plessis, A.J., Evans, A., et al. (2011b): Cerebellar malformations alter regional cerebral development. *Dev. Med. Child Neurol.* **53,** 1128–1134.

Bolduc, M.E., du Plessis, A.J., Sullivan, N., et al. (2012): Regional cerebellar volumes predict functional outcome in children with cerebellar malformations. *Cerebellum* **11,** 531–542.

Boni, S., Valle, G., Cioffi, R.P., et al. (1992): Crossed cerebello-cerebral diaschisis: a SPECT study. *Nucl. Med. Commun.* **13,** 824–831.

Braddock, B.A., Farmer, J.E., Deidrick, K.M., Iverson, J.M. & Maria. B.L. (2006): Oromotor and communication findings in Joubert syndrome: further evidence of multisystem apraxia. *J. Child Neurol.* **21,** 160–163.

Bulgheroni, S., D'Arrigo, S., Valente, E.M. & Riva D. (2014): Cognitive-behavioral phenotype of Joubert syndrome: review of the literature and preliminary data from a project by italian JSRD study group. In: *Paediatric Neurological Disorders with Cerebellar Involvement – Diagnosis and Management,* eds. E.M. Valente & S. D'Arrigo. Mariani Foundation Paediatric Neurology Series, vol. 27. Montrouge: John Libbey, pp. 235–240.

Dror, R., Malinger, G., Ben-Sira, L., Lev, D., Pick, C.G. & Lerman-Sagie, T. (2009): Developmental outcome of children with enlargement of the cisterna magna identified in utero. *J. Child Neurol.* **24,** 1486–1492.

Ecker, J.L., Shipp, T.D., Bromley, B. & Benacerraf. B. (2000): The sonographic diagnosis of Dandy-Walker and Dandy-Walker variant: associated findings and outcomes. *Prenat. Diagn.* **20,** 328–332.

Fennell, E.B., Gitten, J.C., Dede, D.E. & Maria. B.L. (1999): Cognition, behavior, and development in Joubert syndrome. *J. Child Neurol.* **14,** 592–596.

Forzano, F., Mansour, S., Ierullo, A., Homfray, T. & Thilaganathan, B. (2007): Posterior fossa malformation in fetuses: a report of 56 further cases and a review of the literature. *Prenat. Diagn.* **27,** 495–501.

Graf, H., Franke, B. & Abler, B. (2013): Cerebellar cognitive affective syndrome in Dandy-Walker variant disorder. *J. Neuropsych. Clin. Neurosci.* **25,** E45–46.

Gunay-Aygun, M., Parisi, M.A., Doherty, D., et al. (2009): MKS3-related ciliopathy with features of autosomal recessive polycystic kidney disease, nephronophthisis and Joubert syndrome. *J. Pediatr.* **155,** 386–392.

Haimovici, J.A., Doubilet, P.M., Benson, C.B. & Frates, M.C. (1997): Clinical significance of isolated enlargement of the cisterna magna (>10 mm) on prenatal sonography. *J. Ultrasound Med.* **16,** 735–736.

Hodgkins, P.R., Harris, C.M., Shawkat, F.S., *et al.* (2004): Joubert syndrome: long-term follow-up. *Dev. Med. Child Neurol.* **46**, 694–699.

Ito, M. (2008): Control of mental activities by internal models in the cerebellum. *Nat. Rev. Neurosci.* **9**, 304–313.

Klein, O., Pierre-Kahn, A., Boddaert, N., Parisot, D. & Brunelle, F. (2003): Dandy-Walker malformation: prenatal diagnosis and prognosis. *Childs Nerv. Syst.* **19**, 484–489.

Kölble, N., Wisser, J., Kurmanavicius, J., *et al.* (2000): Dandy-walker malformation: prenatal diagnosis and outcome. *Prenat. Diagn.* **20**, 318–327.

Levisohn, L., Cronin-Golomb, A. & Schmahmann, J.D. (2000): Neuropsychological consequences of cerebellar tumour resection in children: cerebellar cognitive affective syndrome in a pediatric population. *Brain* **123**, 1041–1050.

Limperopoulos, C. & du Plessis, A.J. (2006): Disorders of cerebellar growth and development. *Curr. Opin. Pediatr.* **18**, 621–627.

Limperopoulos, C., Robertson, R.L., Estroff, J.A., *et al.* (2006): Diagnosis of inferior vermian hypoplasia by fetal magnetic resonance imaging: potential pitfalls and neurodevelopmental outcome. *Am. J. Obstet. Gynecol.* **194**, 1070–1076.

Long, A., Moran, P. & Robson, S. (2006): Outocome of fetal cerebral posterior fossa anomalies. *Prenat. Diag.* **26**, 707–710.

Maria, B.L., Hoang, K.B., Tusa, R.J., *et al.* (1997): Joubert syndrome revisited: key ocular motor signs with magnetic resonance imaging correlation. *J. Child Neurol.* **12**, 423–430.

Miller, N.G., Reddick, W.E., Kocak, M., *et al.* (2009): Cerebellocerebral diaschisis is the likely mechanism of post-surgical posterior fossa syndrome in pediatric patients with midline cerebellar tumors. *AJNR Am. J. Neuroradiol.* **31**, 288–294.

Morris, E.B., Phillip, N.S., Laningham, F.H., *et al.* (2009): Proximal dentatothalamocortical tract involvement in posterior fossa syndrome. *Brain* **132**, 3087–3095.

Ozonoff, S., Williams, B.J., Gale, S. & Miller, J.N. (1999): Autism and autistic behavior in Joubert syndrome. *J. Child Neurol.* **14**, 636–641.

Poretti, A. (2011): Cognitive functions in children with cerebellar malformations. *Dev. Med. Child Neurol.* **3**, 389.

Poretti, A., Boltshauser, E., Loenneker,T., *et al.* (2007): Diffusion tensor imaging in Joubert syndrome. *AJNR Am. J. Neuroradiol.* **28**, 1929–1933.

Poretti, A., Dietrich Alber, F., Brancati, F., Dallapiccola, B., Valente, E.M. & Boltshauser, E. (2009): Normal cognitive functions in Joubert syndrome. *Neuropediatrics* **40**, 287–290.

Poretti, A., Boltshauser, E. & Doherty, D. (2014): Cerebellar hypoplasia: differential diagnosis and diagnostic approach. *Am. J. Med. Genet. C. Semin. Med. Genet.* **166**, 211–226.

Riva, D., Pantaleoni, C., Nichelli, F., Bulgheroni, S. & Bagnasco, I. (2000): Cerebellum and higher cognitive functions: preliminary results from a sample of children with congenital cerebellar hypoplasia. *Gior. Neuropsich. Età Evol.* **21**, 252–256.

Riva, D. & Giorgi, C. (2000): The cerebellum contributes to higher functions during development: evidence from a series of children surgically treated for posterior fossa tumors. *Brain* **123**, 1051–1061.

Romani, M., Micalizzi, A. & Valente, E.M. (2013): Joubert Syndrome: congenital cerebellar ataxia with the molar tooth. *Lancet Neurol.* **12**, 894–905.

Sasaki-Adams, D., Elbabaa, S.K., Jewells, V., Carter, L., Campbell, J.W. & Ritter, A.M. (2008): The Dandy-Walker variant: a case series of 24 pediatric patients and evaluation of associated anomalies, incidence of hydrocephalus, and developmental outcomes. *J. Neurosurg. Pediatr.* **2**, 194–199.

Schmahmann, J.D. & Sherman, J.C. (1998): The cerebellar cognitive affective syndrome. *Brain* **121**, 561–579.

Steinlin, M., Schmid, M., Landau, K. & Boltshauser, E. (1997): Follow-up in children with Joubert syndrome. *Neuropediatrics* **28**, 204–211.

Steinlin, M., Imfeld, S., Zulauf, P., *et al.* (2003): Neuropsychological long-term sequelae after posterior fossa tumour resection during childhood. *Brain* **126**, 1998–2008.

Takahashi, T.N., Farmer, J.E., Deidrick, K.K., Hsu, B.S., Miles, J.H. & Maria, B.L. (2005): Joubert syndrome is not a cause of classical autism. *Am. J. Med. Genet. A.* **132**, 347–351.

Tarui, T., Limperopoulos, C., Sullivan, N.R., Robertson, R.L. & du Plessis, A.J. (2014): Long-term developmental outcome of children with a fetal diagnosis of isolated inferior vermian hypoplasia. *Arch. Dis. Child Fetal Neonatal Ed.* **99**, 54–58.

Tavano, A. & Borgatti, R. (2010): Evidence for a link among cognition, language and emotion in cerebellar malformations. *Cortex* **46**, 907–918.

Tavano, A., Grasso, R., Gagliardi, C., *et al.* (2007a): Disorders of cognitive and affective development in cerebellar malformations. *Brain* **130,** 2646–2660.

Tavano, A., Fabbro, F. & Borgatti, R. (2007b): Speaking without the cerebellum: language skills in a young adult with near total absence of the cerebellum. In: *Mental States, Evolution, Function, Nature,* eds. Schalley & D. Khlentzos. John Benjamin.

Zimmer, E.Z., Lowenstein, L., Bronshtein, M., Goldsher, D. & Aharon-Peretz, J. (2007): Clinical significance of isolated mega cisterna magna. *Arch. Gynecol. Obstet.* **276,** 487–490.

Chapter 10

Brain tumours: how the location of the lesion and treatments affect cognitive function

Daria Riva, Silvia Esposito, Fabiana Cazzaniga and Sara Bulgheroni

*Developmental Neurology Division, Fondazione IRCCS Istituto Neurologico 'C. Besta',
via Celoria 11, 20133 Milan, Italy*
Daria.Riva@istituto-besta.it

Summary

In parallel with greater interest being devoted to cognitive and emotional deficits secondary to childhood brain tumours, survival rates have risen and surgical, radiation, and medical techniques have improved. Cognitive and behavioural deficits, particularly when chronic, have a marked existential effect, conditioning adolescence and adulthood of patients. The problem is extremely complex as acute or subacute deficits can be distinguished and many intrinsically correlated variables must be considered.

The type and entity of cognitive impairment are associated with three types of risk factors. One set of factors is biological and refers to the type and location of the tumour, as well as to the physiological short- and long-term effects of complementary treatments, including chemotherapy and radiotherapy. A second set of variables is developmental and refers to the chronological age and stage of development of a particular child, and thus to his/her age at diagnosis as well as to the epochs in which treatment and evaluation are carried out. A third set of variables involves "cognitive reserve", defined as pre-illness intelligence, education, and, in particular, constitutional and genetic factors. This variable can prove to be either an advantage or a disadvantage in the recovery of deficits after a brain lesion and accounts for the differences in outcome that are noted in cases when disease stages, types of treatment, and periods of time exposed to therapy appear similar. Extrinsic factors, such as the patient's social environment and the family's lifestyle, can also affect outcome. Psychosocial and environmental factors are now being studied to a greater extent with respect to the past, as they are justifiably considered variables that can improve or aggravate the patient's outcome.

These cognitive and behavioural deficits tend to persist over time in relation to structural brain modifications that have taken place, despite efforts to formulate an individual treatment protocol and the use of sophisticated surgical and radiotherapy techniques. Cognitive rehabilitation needs to be recommended, organized, and implemented, and although only preliminary results are available, they are extremely encouraging.

In conclusion, the cognitive and behavioural outcome in children with brain tumours is the ultimate consequence of an altered developmental trajectory affected by an inextricable set of developmental, biological, and pre-illness constitutional genetic variables. It is important that the neuropsychological and behavioural effects of all these variables be analyzed in the most exhaustive and sophisticated way possible so as to reduce long-term cognitive neurotoxicity.

As survival rates among children treated for brain tumours continue to increase, ever greater interest is being focused on the long-term, late effects of cancer treatment. Brain tumours represent the second most common cancers in paediatric patients; 30 per cent of these form in the posterior fossa compartment and can have significant physical, behavioural, cognitive, and psychosocial long-term effects on children's quality of life. It is in this context that we will outline the neurocognitive outcome of these kinds of tumours (Riva, 2014).

Neurocognitive decline after childhood brain tumours has been associated with three types of risk variables (Dennis *et al.*, 2004; Riva & Giorgi, 2000a):

1. Biological variables are associated with the tumour's location and the physiological effects of adjuvant treatments, such as chemotherapy and/or cranial radiotherapy.

2. Developmental variables are linked to the patient's chronological age and developmental stage, both at the time of diagnosis/treatment and when the final outcome is evaluated.

3. The third set of variables involves *reserve*, which includes pre-diagnosis cognitive and psychosocial resources that buffer or enhance the effect of biological risk. In the case of brain tumours, it is essential to consider *how an individual child might have been if she/he had not been stricken with a tumour*. The pre- and post-diagnosis resources of the child, family, school, and community are all important considerations in this regard.

Biological variables

Biological variables include neurological conditions such as hydrocephalus, tumour localization, surgery, and tumour treatments. *Hydrocephalus* is a significant complication of infratentorial brain tumours (Riva *et al.*, 1994), and up to a third of children with posterior fossa tumours require shunts (Raimondi & Tomita, 1981). Hydrocephalus at the time of tumour treatment does not appear to affect patient outcome, as no correlation has been found between IQ and post-operative ventricular dilation or non-emergency shunt placement (Kao *et al.*, 1994). It is unclear if there is any correlation between shunt history and cognitive outcome.

Structural damage is caused by intracranial pressure and by the length of time pressure has been or is being exerted on brain regions and, in particular, on frontal white matter (Riva *et al.*, 1994; Riva & Giorgi, 2000a; Duffner, 2010).

The roles of *surgery and location* will be discussed later in this section, in which a more detailed description of specific pathological clinical pictures will be outlined.

Radiotherapy

External beam conventional radiotherapy is known to be associated with severe neuropsychological and intellectual deterioration and is thought to involve a progressive vascular demyelinating disorder. As explained above, neurological symptoms present some time after treatment, reach a peak over the next few years, and then a slight, although persistent, decline continues (Cohen & Duffner, 1994). The concomitant cognitive deterioration is inversely correlated to the patient's age at the time of treatment (Packer *et al.*, 1989) and is directly correlated to the dose and the field of cerebral radiation (Mulhern *et al.*, 2004).

The volume of the brain undergoing treatment is an important factor that conditions cognitive outcome. Loss of white matter and/or the failure to develop could partially account for worsening IQ scores, as well as for impairment in non-verbal intelligence, fluency, speed of processing, and executive functions (Fry & Hale, 1996). White matter constitutes the connecting system between the hemispheres and among different brain regions, ensuring the interconnection of the brain system itself. It is thus evident that white matter pathology causes complex neuropsychological malfunctioning caused by the disconnection within cerebral networks.

Technical advances in radiation oncology therapies, such as the development of hyperfractionated radiation therapy, appear to have reduced the frequency and severity of neurocognitive sequelae (Cohen & Duffner, 1994; Riva *et al.*, 1996). Nevertheless, although hyperfractionating radiation doses appear to ensure that healthy tissue will be restored, it has not eliminated the deficits associated with radiotherapy (Riva, 2005). Recent studies have described promising results and preserved cognitive function in children with medulloblastoma 6 years after undergoing hyperfractionated radiation (Gupta *et al.*, 2012). Although so far infrequently utilized for children, new radiotherapeutic techniques such as stereotactic body radiotherapy and brachytherapy appear to be safe and effective and associated with an improvement in long-term neurocognitive outcome.

Chemotherapy

The correlation of *intravenous chemotherapy* with intellectual loss and neuropsychological impairment in children treated for brain tumours is still under discussion. This is due, in part, to the fact that the majority of children are treated with chemotherapy and concomitant cranial radiation. Since neurotoxicity has frequently been found to be associated with cranial radiation in young children with brain tumours, its use is generally postponed. A positive developmental outcome has been reported in very young children treated with chemotherapy alone (Copeland *et al.*, 1999). Cognitive decline over time has been found to be minimal, as demonstrated by nearly normal cognitive, academic, and neuropsychological scores.

The use of *intrathecal chemotherapy*, and, in particular, methotrexate has been correlated with significant cognitive morbidity (Maria *et al.*, 1993), and there appears to be an even greater risk when it is associated with radiotherapy (Bleyer & Poplack, 1985). Although there are few studies focusing entirely on children with medulloblastoma, the literature findings indicate that radiotherapy with intrathecal methotrexate is associated with strongly negative effects on cognitive development (Lesnik *et al.*, 1998; Riva *et al.*, 2002).

The role of surgery and tumour location

The role of surgical intervention is inextricably linked to tumour site. Technologies, procedures, and equipment have made incredible advances in recent years; neuronavigation systems (Giorgi *et al.*, 1989) have made it possible to locate the tumour and to reach it in a precise manner. At the same time, advanced neuroimaging techniques and, in particular, fibre tractography analysis and functional magnetic resonance imaging permit the surgeon to plan the operation in detail and to avoid, or at least limit, damage to the most eloquent brain areas and the white matter bundles. Some surgical procedures, such as the prolonged retraction of the frontal or temporal lobe, the partial sectioning of the corpus callosum to reach tumours of the third ventricle, and the partial incision or destruction of the cerebellar vermis, can lead to specific, critical neuropsychological, as well as behavioural profiles.

Higher cognitive functions are processed by a widely distributed network in the brain involving the participation of many interconnected areas. As a consequence, each area that is damaged contributes to the network's general malfunctioning, as well as to the impaired development of the particular function linked to that specific area. There are, however, some regions (known as "hub nodes") that are more important for processing information and their damage is linked to more serious deficits. It is nevertheless true that every area has its own eloquence and there are no mute areas (Riva, 2011).

Tumours localized in the language areas, the hippocampus, the occipital lobes, and the sellar-suprasellar regions, etc. provoke specific cognitive patterns and specific neuropsychological outcomes. The brain areas most vulnerable to developmental risk, due to the fact that they are not particularly vicarious, comprise: the *basal ganglia*, which are part of largely segregated closed-loop projections proceeding from the basal ganglia to the cortex and from there back again to the basal nuclei; and *the white matter*, the system which ensures the brain's anatomical and functional connectivity and malfunction of which provokes serious short and long-term disturbances in the information circuit.

As tumours of the posterior fossa are the most frequent childhood brain cancers, the cerebellum will be considered separately. The cerebellum, crucial for brain organization, is a particularly relevant associative area also with regard to cognitive development. Two absolutely distinctive syndromes may occur in the event of a lesion. The first is the Cognitive Affective Syndrome, originally described by Schmahmann and Sherman (1998) and later delineated by some studies carried out in children (Levisohn *et al.*, 2000; Riva & Giorgi, 2000b). The syndrome is characterized by cognitive disturbances in the case of hemispheric lesions or by emotional behavioural disturbances due to lesions of the vermis (Schmahmann & Sherman, 1998). Another important specific profile linked to the cerebellum is mutism in children following surgery, more often for a tumour of the posterior fossa rather than for the cerebellar vermis. The mutism noted usually develops within hours or days after removal of a cerebellar tumour and can vary in severity from a dysarthric disorder with good preservation of speech to severe anarthria. The disorder is articulatory and transient, although dysarthria may persist. It was for this reason that it was termed: "cerebellar mutism with subsequent dysarthria" by van Dongen and his collaborators (Vandongen *et al.*, 1994). The disturbance provokes prevalently vascular lesions generally of the vermis or of the deep cerebellar nuclei with bilateral involvement of the dentate nuclei (Ammirati *et al.*, 1989).

Developmental variables

Developmental variables are intrinsically linked to biological variables and include:

1. The age at time of treatment. Brain plasticity decreases with age, but there are some brain regions at greater neurodevelopmental risk than others, among these are the hippocampal and parahippocampal regions and the frontal and cerebellar regions (the frontal-cerebellar system) which are ontogenetically interconnected (Lesnik *et al.*, 1998).

2. The time since treatment. This is also a crucial factor because time permits brain function deficits to be recovered and neuropsychological functions to be redistributed. Some treatments such as radiation therapy are, nevertheless, responsible for progressive neurocognitive and neuropsychological deficits and trigger vascular neuropathological alterations. Deficits frequently present approximately 3 years after therapy has been completed and reach a peak one to 3 years later; afterwards, a less severe but persistent decline continues (Packer *et al.*, 1989).

Cognitive reserve

The third set of variables is correlated to *cognitive reserve and rehabilitation*. Cognitive reserve refers to the brain's ability to maximize performance or to compensate in the face of brain damage; this explains the disparity that has been noted between the degree of brain pathology or damage and its clinical manifestation. Inter-individual diversity is, in fact, very high and extremely different outcomes have been noted in these cases. Cognitive reserve appears to reflect the individual's pre-illness cognitive capacity, genetics, and educational background (Dennis *et al.*, 2000, 2004).

Rehabilitation using a multi-faceted, structured approach that takes into consideration the variables mentioned here is highly recommended not only for motor impairments but also for cognitive and social disorders. Pharmacological therapy, which is often neglected in these cases, also needs to be considered, and not only for depression, which is often reactive to a long history of illness, in an effort to improve the patient's low vitality and functional capacity levels. Metilfenidate may be an appropriate choice (Smithson *et al.*, 2013).

Ecological and environmental interventions involving the patient's family and, at times, psychotherapeutic counselling should also be considered.

In a recent multicentre study, we utilized the International Classification of Functioning, Disability and Health (Vago *et al.*, 2011) to analyze three domains in our patients: communication, daily-life skills, and socialization. The results confirmed that rehabilitation within the context of an enriched socially-active environment, rather than considering only technical aspects (*e.g.* physiotherapy), must be taken into consideration and provided for.

Conclusions

Cognitive deficits are the final outcome of an intrinsic, inextricable convergence of three sets of variables: biological variables linked to the tumour and treatments, developmental variables, and constitutional variables. Surgical interventions are not associated with added deficits when guided properly or when they occur without complications or violation of fundamental structures. Radiotherapy represents a neurodevelopmental risk factor, as do intravenous and intrathecal chemotherapies which can alter neurobiological processes; radiation therapy and chemotherapy can, moreover, cause vasculitis and diffuse white matter changes.

Multidisciplinary examinations by specialists over a long follow-up period, taking into consideration the variables cited, are recommended. This study method has made it possible for us to attain important results because it has permitted us to re-evaluate therapeutic protocols in view of our commitment to finding a balance between survival, which remains a fundamental goal, and the quality of life of our paediatric patients and their families.

Conflicts of interest: none.

References

Ammirati, M., Mirzai, S. & Samii, M. (1989): Transient mutism following removal of a cerebellar tumour. A case report and review of the literature. *Child Nerv. Syst.* **5,** 12–14.

Bleyer, W.A. & Poplack, D.G. (1985): Prophylaxis and treatment of leukemia in the central nervous system and other sanctuaries. *Semin. Oncol.* **12,** 131–148.

Cohen, M.E. & Duffner, P.K. (1994): Long-term clinical effects of radiation and chemotherapy. In: *Brain Tumours in Children*, eds. M.E. Cohen & P.K. Duffner. In: *International review of child neurology. 2nd ed.* pp. 455–481. New York: Raven Press.

Copeland, D.R., deMoor, C., Moore, B.D. & Ater, J.L. (1999): Neurocognitive development of children after a cerebellar tumour in infancy: a longitudinal study. *J. Clin. Oncol.* **17,** 3476–3486.

Dennis, M., Spiegler, B.J. & Hetherington, R. (2000): New survivors for the new millennium: cognitive risk and reserve in adults with childhood brain insults. *Brain Cogn.* **42,** 102–105.

Dennis, M.B., Spiegler, J., Riva, D., Daune, L. & MacGregor, D.L. (2004): Neuropsychological outcome. In: *Brain and Spinal Tumours of Childhood,* eds. D. Walker, G. Perilongo, R. Taylor & J. Punt. pp. 213–227. Routledge.

Duffner, P.K. (2010): Risk factors for cognitive decline in children treated for brain tumours. *Eur. J. Paediatr. Neurol.* **14,** 106–115.

Fry, A.S. & Hale, S. (1996): Processing speed, working memory, and fluid intelligence: evidence for a developmental cascade. *Psychol. Sci,* **4,** 237–241.

Giorgi, C., Broggi, G., Casolino, D., Franzini, A. & Pluchino, F. (1989): Computer-assisted analysis of neuroradiological data in planning neurosurgical procedures. *J. Neurosurg. Sci.* **33,** 19–22.

Gupta, T., Jalali, R., Goswami, S., et al. (2012): Early clinical outcomes demonstrate preserved cognitive function in children with average-risk medulloblastoma when treated with hyperfractionated radiation therapy. *Int. J. Radiat. Oncol. Biol. Phys.* **83,** 1534–1540.

Kao, G.D., Goldwein, J.W., Schultz, D.J., Radcliffe, J., Sutton, L. & Lange, B. (1994): The impact of perioperative factors on subsequent intelligence quotient deficits in children treated for medulloblastoma posterior-fossa primitive neuroectodermal tumours. *Cancer* **74,** 965–971.

Lesnik, P.G., Ciesielski, K.T., Hart, B.L., Benzel, E.C. & Sanders, J.A. (1998): Evidence for cerebellar-frontal subsystem changes in children treated with intrathecal chemotherapy for leukemia- enhanced data analysis using an effect size model. *Arch. Neurol.* **55,** 1561–1568.

Levisohn, L., Cronin-Golomb, A. & Schmahmann, J.D. (2000): Neuropsychological consequences of cerebellar tumour resection in children- cerebellar cognitive affective syndrome in a paediatric population. *Brain* **123,** 1041–1050.

Maria, B.L., Dennis, M. & Obonsawin, M. (1993): Severe permanent encephalopathy in acute lymphoblastic-leukemia. *Canad. J. Neurol. Sciences* **20,** 199–205.

Mulhern, R., Merchant, T., Gajjar, A., Reddick, W. & Kun, L. (2004): Late neurocognitive sequelae in survivors of brain tumours in childhood. *Lancet Oncol.* **5,** 399–408.

Packer, R.J., Sutton, L.N., Atkins, et al. (1989): A prospective study of cognitive function in children receiving whole-brain radiotherapy and chemotherapy: 2-year results. *J. Neurosurg.* **70,** 707–713.

Raimondi, A.J. & Tomita, T. (1981): Hydrocephalus and infratentorial tumours. Incidence, clinical picture, and treatment. *J. Neurosurg.* **55,** 174–182.

Riva, D. (2005): Individuazione di criteri prognostici neuropsicologici nella scelta del trattamento dei tumouri cerebrali infantili. Relazione della Ricerca Triennale finanziata dal Ministero della Sanità. Rome.

Riva, D. (2011): Higher cognitive function processing in developmental age: specialized areas, connections, and distributed networks. In: *Brain Lesion Localization and Developmental Functions,* eds. D. Riva, C. Njiokiktjien & S. Bulgheroni, pp. 1–8. Mariani Foundation Paediatric Neurology Series, vol. 25. John Libbey Eurotext.

Riva, D. (2014): Medulloblastoma in developmental age: long-term neurocognitive and emotional-behavioral outcome. In: *The Medulloblastoma Dook,* eds. D. Kombogiorgas, pp. 207–216. Nova Science Publishers.

Riva, D. & Giorgi, C. (2000a): The neurodevelopmental price of survival in children with malignant brain tumours. *Child Nerv. Syst.* **16,** 751–754.

Riva, D. & Giorgi, C. (2000b): The cerebellum contributes to higher functions during development- evidence from a series of children surgically treated for posterior fossa tumours. *Brain* **123,** 1055–1061.

Riva, D., Milani, N., Giorgi, C., Pantaleoni, C., Zorzi, C. & Devoti, M. (1994): Intelligence outcome in children with shunted hydrocephalus of different etiology. *Child Nerv. Syst.* **10,** 70–73.

Riva, D., Milani, N., Pantaleoni, C., Devoti, M. & Giorgi, C. (1996): New techniques for treatments of brain tumours in children: the neuropsychological outcome. *J. Int. Neuropsychol. Soc.* **12,** 412.

Riva, D., Giorgi, C., Nichelli, F., et al. (2002): Intrathecal methotrexate affects cognitive function in children with medulloblastoma. *Neurology* **59,** 48–53.

Schmahmann, J.D. & Sherman, J.C. (1998): The cerebellar cognitive affective syndrome. *Brain* **121,** 561–579.

Smithson, E.F., Phillips, R., Harvey, D.W. & Morrall, M.C. (2013): The use of stimulant medication to improve neurocognitive and learning outcomes in children diagnosed with brain tumours: a systematic review. *Eur. J. Cancer* **49,** 3029–3040.

Vago, C., Bulgheroni, S., Usilla, A., et al. (2011): Adaptive functioning in children in the first six months after surgery for brain tumours. *Disabil. Rehabil.* **33,** 953–960.

Vandongen, H.R., Catsmanberrevoets, C.E. & Vanmourik, M. (1994): The syndrome of brain cerebellar mutism and subsequent dysarthria. *Neurology* **44,** 2040–2046.

Chapter 11

Paediatric anaesthetic and cognitive neurotoxicity

Lena S. Sun

*Depts. of Anesthesiology and Paediatrics, Columbia University Medical Center,
CH 4-440 North, 622 West 168th Street, New York 10032, USA*
lss4@cumc.columbia.edu

Summary

In the developing brain of rodents and non-human primates, commonly used anaesthetic agents (acting as GABA receptor agonists and/or NMDA receptor antagonists) have been documented to induce neuroapoptosis, neurodegeneration, impaired neurogenesis, and other cellular effects. Adult animals that had early life anaesthesia exposure have been shown to have persistent neurobehavioural and functional deficits including abnormal behaviour, attention, learning and memory tasks, as well as social behaviour. Clinical studies to assess neurodevelopmental outcome have been conducted in premature infants and children undergoing congenital cardiac surgery, craniosynostosis surgery, eye surgery, and minor surgical procedures (*e.g.* hernia). The results have been conflicting with respect to the long-term neurodevelopmental outcome following surgery and early anaesthesia exposure. While a number of retrospective cohort clinical studies have found that young children exposed to anaesthesia have an increased risk of learning disability, developmental delay, behaviour disorders, autism-spectrum disorders, and poor academic performance, other studies have reported that academic school performance and behaviour were unaffected by anaesthesia exposure. Further research will be needed to better define the neurodevelopmental safety of anaesthesia in young children.

Introduction

The safety of anaesthesia in infants and children has become a serious concern due to mounting and convincing evidence from pre-clinical studies that anaesthetics in common clinical use are neurotoxic to the developing brain and cause long-term neurobehavioural abnormalities. However, clinical data are much more inconclusive. We will review data from published clinical studies that have examined neurodevelopmental outcome in children who had surgery and anaesthesia. We will also present some of the ongoing studies related to anaesthesia and cognitive neurotoxicity in children.

Table 2. Summary of clinical studies: risks of abnormal neurocognitive effects after early childhood anesthesia exposure

Increased risk	No increased risk
Wilder et al. (multiple exposure)	Wilder et al. (single exposure)
Flick et al. (multiple exposure)	Flick et al. (single exposure)
Sprung et al. (multiple exposure)	Sprung et al. (single exposure)
Di Maggio et al. (2009)	Hansen et al. (2011)
Di Maggio et al. (2011)	Hansen et al. (2013)
Naumann et al.	Guerra et al. (2011)
Ing et al.	Fan et al.
Block et al.	Roze et al.
Guerra et al. (2013)	Chorne et al.
Kabra et al.	Filan et al.
Hintz et al.	
Elsinga et al.	
Bong et al.	

associated with a significant greater risk of having one or more neurosensory impairment. This study examined a total of 426 infants with birth weights between 500 to 999 grams, who had symptomatic PDA (Kabra et al., 2007); 110 underwent surgery for ligation of PDA, and 316 received indomethacin as medical therapy. There were no differences in death rate between the surgical and medical groups; 13.6 per cent or 15 children in the surgical group and 22.5 per cent or 71 children in the medical therapy group died. However, among the survivors, the surgical group had a higher risk of one or more neurosensory impairment compared to the medical group (50/95 in the surgical group and 84/245 in the medical group). A single centre study from the University of California at San Francisco (UCSF) consisted of a total cohort of 446 infants with < 28 weeks gestational age who had PDA (Chorne et al., 2007). The study assessed the outcome of neonatal comorbidities (including retinopathy of prematurity, necrotizing enterocolitis, chronic lung disease, and neurodevelopmental impairment) associated with PDA in surgically and medically managed patients. Surgical PDA ligation was found to be significantly and independently associated with an increased incidence of chronic lung disease, independent of an infant's gestational age or other PDA-related variables. However, in contrast to the TIPP results, surgical ligation did not increase the risk of adverse neurodevelopmental outcome.

Exploratory laparotomy

Neurodevelopmental outcome has also been studied in premature infants undergoing exploratory laparotomy for necrotizing enterocolitis (NEC) and other bowel surgeries. Using the VLBW (Very Low Birth Weight) Registry as the data source, surgically-treated infants (< 1,000 grams birth weight) with necrotizing enterocolitis were found to be at higher risk of adverse neurodevelopmental outcome compared to those who had only been medically treated (Hintz et al., 2005). This study had a total of 4,933 infants. The study subjects were divided into three groups based on the diagnosis and management of necrotizing enterocolitis (NEC): (1) no NEC (2,703 survivors completed follow-up); (2) medically-treated NEC (124 survivors completed follow-up); and (3) surgically-treated NEC (121 survivors completed follow-up). Their neurodevelopment outcomes were assessed at 18-22 months corrected age using Bayley Scale-II. The surgically-treated NEC group was found to have increased risk of low scores in Mental Development Index, Psychomotor Development Index, and Neurodevelopment Impairment compared to the other two groups. Filan and colleagues (2012) studied premature infants (< 30 weeks gestational age or < 1,250 grams of birth weight) who had surgery requiring general anaesthesia during the neonatal period (bowel surgery, inguinal hernia, and PDA ligation; total $n = 30$) and assessed the infants at a comparable age. They found neonatal surgery and general anaesthesia did not increase the risk of impaired cognitive outcome. This study compared surgically-treated premature neonates with non-surgical controls ($n = 178$). The surgical group was found to have greater white matter injury and smaller total brain volumes at age 2 years but not worse cognitive outcomes. Elsinga and collaborators (2013) studied a cohort of Neonatal Intensive Care Unit (NICU) infants (total $n = 27$) who had laparotomy for intestinal obstruction, and found them to have an increased risk of poor motor function and deficits in selective attention when compared to the normal population. The study focused on only infants who had surgery and anaesthesia for intestinal obstruction. Unlike the two studies cited above (Filan et al., 2012; Hintz et al., 2005), the age at assessment of neurocognitive functions of this study cohort was much later (6-13 years). Taken together, these studies thus do not provide conclusive evidence with regard to whether surgery/anaesthesia in premature and low-birth-weight infants could be associated with an increased risk of neurodevelopmental impairment.

Paediatric surgical patients

Neurodevelopmental outcome studies have been conducted in a variety of paediatric surgical cohorts, including those who underwent 'minor' infant surgery, congenital heart surgery, craniosynostosis surgery, and eye surgery. Some of these studies have examined specific types of surgical procedures, while others have included a wide range of surgical procedures.

Several studies have specifically examined the outcome in inguinal hernia patients. Di Maggio and colleagues (2009) created a birth cohort including all children enrolled in the New York State Medicaid from 1999 to 2001. The authors used the ICD-9 code for inguinal hernia surgery before age 36 months as the exposure variable, and the diagnostic codes for developmental delay, intellectual disability, autism spectrum disorders, speech/language problems, and behaviour problems as the outcome variable. Confounding variables included in the analysis were low birth weight, perinatal hypoxia, perinatal infections, and CNS anomalies. For comparison, the authors used a group derived from random sampling, matched for age, who did not have the procedure code for inguinal hernia surgery. Their conclusion was that inguinal hernia surgery and anaesthesia was associated with an increased risk of developmental and behavioural disorders. Hansen and collaborators (2011) conducted a birth cohort study in infants exposed to anaesthesia during inguinal hernia surgery using the Danish National Patient Register (1986-1990). This study used a random age-matched 5 per cent population sample as the comparison group. The primary outcome was the ninth grade test scores and teachers' scores. Although no difference in primary outcome was found, there was a significant difference between groups in the secondary outcome, defined as 'non-attainment of score'. Inguinal hernia (with or without orchiopexy) was one of the three surgical procedures in the study from the University of Iowa (Block et al., 2012). This study examined infants (under age 1 year) who had one of the three following surgeries: inguinal hernia with or without orchiopexy, pyloromyotomy, or circumcision (Block *et al.*, 2012). The outcome measure used was the composite score on the Iowa Tests of Basic Skills and Educational Development (IOWA test scores). The authors examined both the mean scores and the proportion of the group that scored in the lowest 5 per cent, in comparison to the population norm. From the initial total of 519 subjects whose relevant medical records were retrievable, Group 1 consisted of those who had available IOWA test scores ($n = 287$). Group 2 were those who responded and agreed to participate from Group 1 and totalled 133. The authors applied a list of 18 pre-specified CNS-related problems or risk factors to Group 2, and 58 subjects were found to have none of these risk factors and made up Group 3. In both Groups 1 and 2, the mean scores were significantly lower than the population mean, but not in Group 3. However, in all three groups, there was a disproportionally larger percentage of the group that scored within the lower 5 per cent of the IOWA tests (12 per cent in Group 1, 11 per cent in Group 2, and 14 per cent in Group 3). The authors concluded that anaesthesia and surgery during infancy was associated with an over-representation of low IOWA test scores. Similarly, inguinal hernia surgery was among the 'minor infant surgery' examined in the study by Bong and colleagues (2013). They used a case-control design, matching 100 healthy children in Singapore who had minor surgery (inguinal hernias, circumcisions, cystoscopies, and pyloromyotomies) under general anaesthesia before age 1 year with 106 age-matched children without anaesthesia or sedation exposure, and outcomes were assessed at age 12 years. Two different outcome measures were used: (1) academic performance using the standardized aggregate PSLE scores and (2) diagnosis of learning disability. Their conclusion was that anaesthesia during infancy did not have any effect on academic performance but increased the risk of learning disability. It is worth noting that in the studies above, in which an increased risk of adverse neurodevelopmental outcome was found, this occurred with either single or multiple episodes of surgery/anaesthesia.

Hansen and collaborators (2013) also used the Danish National Patient Register (1986-1990) to examine academic performance in infants under three months of age who were exposed to anaesthesia during pyloromyotomy, and compared them to a random age-matched 5 per cent population sample, using ninth grade test scores and teachers' scores as the primary outcome. Their results were similar to findings from those who had inguinal hernia surgery before age 1 year.

The neurodevelopmental effects of anaesthesia exposure in craniosynostosis surgical patients were specifically analyzed by Naumann and colleagues (2012). using the data from a longitudinal neurodevelopmental outcome study in children with single suture craniosynostosis. The study cohort consisted of a total of 70 infants with single suture craniosynostosis surgery who received sevoflurane and/or isoflurane for anaesthesia before age six months. Neurodevelopmental outcome was assessed at age 36 months using the Bayley-II and Preschool Language Test. Analyses were adjusted for types of suture and age at surgery. The results demonstrated an inversely related association between neurodevelopmental scores and the duration of surgery/anaesthesia.

A study conducted in China examined a group of children who had general sevoflurane anaesthesia for strabismus surgery between ages 4 and 7 years ($n = 72$) (Fan *et al.*, 2013). The average duration of exposure was about 1 hour. The authors examined serial IQ tests as a means to assess cognitive function at three different time points; before surgery and at 1 and 6 months after surgery. The results in this much older group of children found no decrease in IQ post-sevoflurane anaesthesia. It is interesting to note that, in fact, there was an increase in IQ in these children.

Several epidemiological studies have examined the effects of anaesthesia exposure in a more mixed surgical group of children.

There were a total of three studies that examined the effects of early childhood exposure using the Olmsted County birth cohort from 1976 to 1982 (a fourth study focusing on examining prenatal anaesthesia exposure will not be detailed here). Two of the studies used 'learning disability' as the outcome parameter. A positive finding for learning disability was defined as learning disability in reading or verbal language or mathematics. The first study comprised a total of 539 children undergoing a total of 875 procedures, who required general anaesthesia before age 4 years (Wilder *et al.*, 2009). The anaesthetics used were predominantly halothane and nitrous (88 per cent had halothane, 91 per cent had nitrous oxide), and ketamine was used in most of the remaining cases (9 per cent received ketamine). The authors reported an increased risk of learning disability for multiple, but not single, anaesthetic exposure. To further determine whether the frequency of exposure may be a consequence of the health status of the child, the authors used the same cohort in a second study but conducted a case control study in the subgroup who had procedure and general anaesthesia prior to age 2 years (Flick *et al.*, 2011). They used two methods for adjustment for health status: the ASA Physical Status assignment and the Hopkins ACG case mix system. Their results were the same as in the first study, showing that multiple, but not single, anaesthesia exposure was associated with an increased risk of learning disability. In addition, there was also a demonstrable need for language IEP. The third study using the same cohort found multiple, but not single, anaesthesia exposure before age 2 years increased the risk of ADHD (Attention Deficit Hyperactivity Disorder) (Sprung *et al.*, 2012). A second study by Di Maggio and collaborators (2011) used a birth cohort of twin births from the NYS Medicaid dataset (1999-2005). Any child was considered to have exposure to anaesthesia if there was an ICD-9 procedure code for any type of surgery before age 36 months, and included in the analysis if there was no history of developmental disorder. ICD-9 diagnostic codes for developmental delay, intellectual disability, autism spectrum disorders, speech/language problems, and behaviour problems were used as the outcome variable. Confounding variables included in the analysis were low birth weight, perinatal hypoxia, perinatal infections, and CNS anomalies. The study found that anaesthesia and surgery before age three years was associated with an increased risk of subsequent diagnosis of developmental or behaviour disorders.

Using the Young Netherlands Twin Registry, Bartels and colleagues (2009) two different outcomes: education achievement (using standardized achievement scores) and cognitive problems (identified using the Conners' Teacher's short form). They questioned the parents with regard to whether their children had received anaesthesia both before age 3 years and age 12 years. The twins in the registry were divided into three groups: twins who were concordant for exposure to anaesthesia, at age 3 years or 12 years; twins who were concordant for no anaesthesia exposure before age 12 years; and twins who were discordant for anaesthesia exposure before age 3 years or 12 years. The results of their analysis found there were no differences in outcome in twins who were discordant for exposure. Interestingly, the concordant unexposed twins had more favourable outcome compared to both of the other two groups, thus suggesting anaesthesia exposure may be a marker for vulnerability and not the cause for adverse neurodevelopmental outcome.

The Western Australian Pregnancy or Raine cohort consists of 2,900 pregnant women in their early pregnancy. The Raine birth cohort includes 2,868 children born to these mothers. The health and other related data regarding these children have been reviewed in detail on eleven occasions at ages 1, 2, 3, 5, 8, 10, 14, 17, 18, 20, and now at 23 years of age. Direct neuropsycholgical tests and parental interviews were performed at these different ages. The largest number of tests was performed at age 10 years, and they included testing for cognitive function (using Symbol Digit Modality Test or SDMT and Raven's Colored Progressive Matrices or CPM), language (using Clinical Evaluation of Language Fundamentals or CELF and Peabody Picture Vocabulary or PPCT), and motor function (using McCarron Assessment of Neuromuscular Development or MAND), with reports of behaviour (using Child Behavior Checklist or CBCL). A total of 2,608 children were included in the analysis for age 10 years. They were divided into an exposed cohort, those who had surgery/anaesthesia before age 3 years ($n = 321$), and those who did not ($n = 2,287$) (Ing et al., 2012), and adjusted for family income, maternal education, and birth weight. The exposed cohort had significantly lower scores in language, both receptive and expressive, and total, as well as in abstract reasoning, but not in all other neuropsychological domains or in behaviour. Therefore, anaesthesia exposure before age 3 years was associated with impaired language and abstract reasoning. This was found with either single or multiple episodes of anaesthesia exposure, at variance with the findings from the Olmsted County analysis.

Neurodevelopmental outcome studies in paediatric patients receiving sedation/analgesia

In pre-clinical studies, the dose and duration of anaesthetic exposure appeared to significantly influence the neurocognitive effects of the exposure. However, only a limited number of studies have focused on the neurodevelopmental outcome in paediatric patients who received prolonged sedation and analgesia.

In a study of the Epipage cohort, the prolonged use of sedation and analgesia in neonates in the Neonatal Intensive Care Unit (NICU) was shown to not increase the risk of neurodevelopmental impairment. The study was conducted for a total of 1,572 premature infants between 22 to 32 weeks of gestational age who had received mechanical ventilation, and neuropsychological assessment was performed using the Kaufman Assessment battery. Comparing the 115 who had prolonged exposure to sedation and/or analgesia with 1,457 who did not, after adjustment using a propensity score as well as for gestational age, neurological outcome at age 5 years was unaffected by prolonged sedation and/or analgesia (Rozé et al., 2008).

The neurodevelopmental outcome of perioperative sedation/analgesia has been specifically investigated by the Western Canadian Complex Paediatric Therapies Follow-Up Group. The study cohort consists of children who had congenital cardiac surgery before age six weeks. Their first study ($n = 95$) assessed the neurodevelopmental outcome at age 18-24 months using Bayley II or III and the General Adaptive Composite (GAC) and the motor scores of the Adaptive Behavior and Assessment System (GAC of ABASA-II) to evaluate mental, motor or vocabulary delay and adaptive skills (Guerra et al., 2011). They collected data on sedation/analgesia retrospectively, and calculated for each drug class (inhaled anaesthetic, opioids, benzodiazepines, ketamine, and chloral hydrate) the total dose, daily average dose, and total number of days. They found no association between sedation/analgesia and neurodevelopmental outcome. Their second study ($n = 91$) conducted the outcome assessment at kindergarten age (Garcia Guerra et al., 2014). In addition to the two assessment instruments used in the first study, they also used a test for visual motor integration (VMI-V). Their results found that there was a significant association between total days of chloral hydrate use and performance IQ, and the total dose of benzodiazepines was associated with a lower visual integration score. These two studies in the same cohort conducted at two different ages underscore the need to perform longitudinal follow-up in vulnerable patients at different stages of brain and neurodevelopment.

In summary, all of the studies, to date, have been almost entirely retrospective in nature. These studies have examined children who had exposure to anaesthesia at different ages, with and without a variety of co-existing medical conditions and with exposure to inhaled and other anaesthetic/sedative agents. The outcomes that were assessed were extremely diverse, from cognitive outcomes, assessed using neuropsychological instruments and diagnoses of learning disability, developmental disorders or attention disorders, scholastic outcomes, using standardized academic achievement testing, and behavioural outcomes, through parent reporting or by clinical diagnoses.

Ongoing studies in anaesthesia and neurodevelopment

There are three ongoing studies that are specifically designed to address the issue of the neurodevelopmental risk of early childhood exposure. These three studies are the GAS study, the PAND study, and the MASK study. The GAS study is a study recruiting from multiple international sites including Australia, Canada, Italy, UK, and USA. The GAS study is a randomized controlled trial with a total sample size of 720 that will be randomized to either a sevoflurane anaesthesia or regional anaesthesia in infants under 60 weeks, post-conceptual age, undergoing inguinal hernia surgery. All of the study subjects will have complete neuropsychological assessment at age 2 years and 5 years.

The Paediatric Anaesthesia NeuroDevelopment Assessment (PANDA) study is an ambi-directional cohort study using a sibling comparison group. The study compares ASA physical status 1 or 2 children who had a single episode of general anaesthesia for inguinal hernia surgery at age 36 months or before with their siblings who had no anaesthesia or sedation before age 36 months. The assessment is performed in both siblings using a comprehensive neuropsychological battery at age between 8 to 15 years (Sun, 2010).

The Mayo Anaesthesia Kids Study (MASK) uses a similar ambi-directional study design. The study will comprise children who had general anaesthesia before age 3 years, either as a single episode of exposure or with multiple episodes of exposure. The control group will be a propensity age-matched group. Testing of the study subjects will occur either at ages between 7-11 or between 15-19. The neuropsychological battery will include the Operant Test Battery that was used in the non-primate study.

A summary of these three ongoing studies is presented in *Table 3*, including the timeline for the completion of these studies.

Table 3. Summary of ongoing studies

	Study Design	Sample size	Age of exposure	Ages of assessment	Comparison group(s)	Addresses neurocognitive risks	Recruitment complete	Assessment complete	Results available
GAS	RCT	720	≤ 1 year	2 and 5 years	GA vs. RA	GA vs. RA Single procedure	2013	2017	2017
PANDA	Ambi-directional	200	0-3 years	8-15 years	Sibling comparison	Single GA ASA 1 and 2	2013-14	2014	2014-15
MASK	Ambi-directional	1,000	0-3 years	7-11 years 15-19 years	Propensity-matched control group	Single & multiple GA	2016	2016	2016

Conclusions

Based on the available study results, there is currently insufficient and inadequate evidence to support any changes in clinical practice of paediatric anaesthesia. These ongoing studies will likely provide more specific outcome data related to the effects of early childhood anaesthesia exposure, and possibly guidance in future practices of anaesthesia in the very young.

Conflicts of interest: none.

References

Bartels, M., Althoff, R.R. & Boomsma, D.I. (2009): Anaesthesia and cognitive performance in children: no evidence for a causal relationship. *Twin Res. Hum. Genet.* **12,** 246–253.

Block, R.I., Thomas, J.J., Bayman, E.O., Choi, J.Y., Kimble, K.K. & Todd, M.M. (2012): Are anaesthesia and surgery during infancy associated with altered academic performance during childhood? *Anesthesiology* **117,** 494–503.

Bong, C.L., Allen, J.C. & Kim, J.T. (2013): The effects of exposure to general anaesthesia in infancy on academic performance at age 12. *Anesth. Analg.* **117,** 1419–1428.

Chorne, N., Leonard, C., Piecuch, R. & Clyman, R.I. (2007): Patent ductus arteriosus and its treatment as risk factors for neonatal and neurodevelopmental morbidity. *Paediatrics* **119,** 1165–1174.

Di Maggio, C., Sun, L.S., Kakavouli, A., Byrne, M.W. & Li, G. (2009): A retrospective cohort study of the association of anaesthesia and hernia repair surgery with behavioral and developmental disorders in young children. *J. Neurosurg. Anesthesiol.* **21,** 286–291.

Di Maggio, C., Sun, L.S. & Li, G. (2011): Early childhood exposure to anaesthesia and risk of developmental and behavioral disorders in a sibling birth cohort. *Anesth. Analg.* **113,** 1143–1151.

Elsinga, R.M., Roze, E., Van Braeckel, K.N., Hulscher, J.B. & Bos, A.F. (2013): Motor and cognitive outcome at school age of children with surgically treated intestinal obstructions in the neonatal period. *Early Hum. Dev.* **89**(3), 181–185.

Fan, Q., Cai, Y., Chen, K. & Li, W. (2013): Prognostic study of sevoflurane-based general anaesthesia on cognitive function in children. *J. Anesth.* **27,** 493–439.

Filan, P.M., Hunt, R.W., Anderson, P.J., Doyle, L.W. & Inder, T.E. (2012): Neurologic outcomes in very preterm infants undergoing surgery. *J. Pediatr.* **160,** 409–414.

Flick, R.P., Katusic, S.K., Colligan, R.C., et al. (2011): Cognitive and behavioral outcomes after early exposure to anaesthesia and surgery. *Paediatrics* **128,** e1053–1061.

Fredriksson, A., Pontén, E., Gordh, T. & Eriksson, P. (2007): Neonatal exposure to a combination of N-methyl-D-aspartate and gamma-aminobutyric acid type A receptor anaesthetic agents potentiates apoptotic neurodegeneration and persistent behavioral deficits. *Anesthesiology* **107,** 427–436.

Garcia Guerra, G., Robertson, C.M., Alton, G.Y., et al.; Western Canadian Complex Pediatric Therapies Follow-up Group. (2014): Neurotoxicity of sedative and analgesia drugs in young infants with congenital heart disease: 4-year follow-up. *Paediatr. Anaesth.* **24,** 257–265.

Guerra, G.G., Robertson, C.M., Alton, G.Y., et al.; Western Canadian Complex Pediatric Therapies Follow-up Group. (2011): Neurodevelopmental outcome following exposure to sedative and analgesic drugs for complex cardiac surgery in infancy. *Paediatr. Anaesth.* **21,** 932–941.

Hansen, T.G., Pedersen, J.K., Henneberg, S.W., et al. (2011): Academic performance in adolescence after inguinal hernia repair in infancy: a nationwide cohort study. *Anesthesiology* **114**(5), 1076–1085.

Hansen, T.G., Pedersen, J.K., Henneberg, S.W., Morton, N.S. & Christensen, K. (2013): Educational outcome in adolescence following pyloric stenosis repair before 3 months of age: a nationwide cohort study. *Paediatr. Anaesth.* **23,** 883–890.

Head, B.P., Patel, H.H., Niesman, I.R., Drummond, J.C., Roth, D.M. & Patel, P.M. (2009): Inhibition of p75 neurotrophin receptor attenuates isoflurane-mediated neuronal apoptosis in the neonatal central nervous system. *Anesthesiology* **110,** 813–825.

Hintz, S.R., Kendrick, D.E., Stoll, B.J., et al.; NICHD Neonatal Research Network. (2005): Neurodevelopmental and growth outcomes of extremely low birth weight infants after necrotizing enterocolitis. *Paediatrics* **115,** 696-703.

Ing, C., Di Maggio, C., Whitehouse, A., et al. (2012): Long-term differences in language and cognitive function after childhood exposure to anaesthesia. *Paediatrics* **130,** e476–485.

Jevtovic-Todorovic, V., Hartman, R.E., Izumi, Y., et al. (2003a): Early exposure to common anaesthetic agents causes widespread neurodegeneration in the developing rat brain and persistent learning deficits. *J. Neurosci.* **23,** 876–882.

Jevtovic-Todorovic, V., Beals, J., Benshoff, N. & Olney, J.W. (2003b): Prolonged exposure to inhalational anaesthetic nitrous oxide kills neurons in adult rat brain. *Neuroscience* **122**(3), 609–616.

Kabra, N.S., Beals, J., Benshoff, N. & Olney, J.W. (2007): Neurosensory impairment after surgical closure of patent ductus arteriosus in extremely low birth weight infants: results from the Trial of Indomethacin Prophylaxis in Preterms. *J. Pediatr.* **150,** 229–234.

Mellon, R.D., Simone, A.F. & Rappaport, B.A. (2007): Use of anaesthetic agents in neonates and young children. *Anesth. Analg.* **104,** 509–520.

Mintz, C.D., Smith, S.C., Barrett, K.M. & Benson, D.L. (2012): Anaesthetics interfere with the polarization of developing cortical neurons. *J. Neurosurg. Anesthesiol.* **24,** 368–375.

Mintz, C.D., Barrett, K.M., Smith, S.C., Benson, D.L. & Harrison, N.L. (2013): Anaesthetics interfere with axon guidance in developing mouse neocortical neurons in vitro via a gamma-aminobutyric acid type A receptor mechanism. *Anesthesiology* **118,** 825–833.

Naumann, H.L., Haberkern, C.M., Pietila, K.E., et al. (2012): Duration of exposure to cranial vault surgery: associations with neurodevelopment among children with single-suture craniosynostosis. *Paediatr. Anaesth.* [Epub ahead of print].

Paule, M.G., Li, M., Allen, R.R., et al. (2011): Ketamine anaesthesia during the first week of life can cause long-lasting cognitive deficits in rhesus monkeys. *Neurotoxicol. Teratol.* **33,** 220–230.

Pearn, M.L., Hu, Y., Niesman, I.R., et al. (2012): Propofol neurotoxicity is mediated by p75 neurotrophin receptor activation. *Anesthesiology* **116,** 352–361.

Rothstein, S., Simkins, T. & Nunez, J.L. (2008): Response to neonatal anaesthesia: effect of sex on anatomical and behavioral outcome. *Neuroscience* **152,** 959–969.

Rozé, J.C., Denizot, S., Carbajal, R., et al. (2008): Prolonged sedation and/or analgesia and 5-year neurodevelopment outcome in very preterm infants: results from the EPIPAGE cohort. *Arch. Pediatr. Adolesc. Med.* **162,** 728–733.

Sanders, R.D., Xu, J., Shu, Y., et al. (2009): Dexmedetomidine attenuates isoflurane-induced neurocognitive impairment in neonatal rats. *Anesthesiology* **110,** 1077–1085.

Sprung, J., Flick, R.P., Katusic, S.K., et al. (2012): Attention-deficit/hyperactivity disorder after early exposure to procedures requiring general anaesthesia. *Mayo Clin. Proc.* **87,** 120–129.

Stratmann, G., Sall, J.W., May, L.D., et al. (2009): Isoflurane differentially affects neurogenesis and long-term neurocognitive function in 60-day-old and 7-day-old rats. *Anesthesiology* **110,** 834–848.

Sun, L. (2010): Early childhood general anaesthesia exposure and neurocognitive development. *Br. J. Anaesth.* **105,** i61–68.

Wilder, R.T., Flick, R.P., Sprung, J., et al. (2009): Early exposure to anaesthesia and learning disabilities in a population-based birth cohort. *Anesthesiology* **110,** 796–804.

Zhu, C., Gao, J., Karlsson, N., et al. (2010): Isoflurane anaesthesia induced persistent, progressive memory impairment, caused a loss of neural stem cells, and reduced neurogenesis in young, but not adult, rodents. *J. Cereb. Blood Flow Metab.* **30,** 1017–1030.

Neurodevelopmental disorders

in general mental abilities, at least one domain of adaptive functioning (conceptual, social, or practical) should be sufficiently impaired for ongoing support to be needed in order for the person to perform adequately in one or more life settings at school, work, or home, or in the community.

Concerning cognitive development, ID can be extremely heterogeneous. It is important to remember that despite a common diagnosis of ID, a "classic" cognitive phenotype may not occur in all affected individuals and several differences also within the same domain may occur, with areas of strength and weakness (Vicari et al., 2004). Different cognitive profiles exhibited by the various aetiological groups of people with ID have been related to the specific characteristics of their genotype as well as to anomalous brain development (Menghini et al., 2011a, 2011b).

Review of the topic

In the last few years, several neuropsychological studies have allowed us to define different cognitive phenotypes related to the brain and genotypes of children with ID, particularly in individuals with genetic syndromes. Two lines of thought have been outlined over time, corresponding to a conceptual evolutionary hypothesis and another purely structural hypothesis. According to the first hypothesis, the cognitive profile of individuals with ID would be characterized by a curve of slowed development comparable to that of a child under the age of typical development ("Developmental lag hypothesis", Zigler & Balla, 1982). In the second hypothesis, instead, the difference between individuals typically developing and those with ID is attributed to a structural organization of cognition which is qualitatively different, where the general principles have different properties for each of the two cases ("Structural lag hypothesis"; Ellis et al., 1982). This contraposition between developmental and structural evolution has in fact been succeeded, since it is now believed that both components play a role in this process. Thus, in ID, development of different cognitive functions could be considered as delayed and incomplete, but also atypical and qualitatively different. This concept might be well suited to genetic syndromes in which it is impossible to draw a uniform cognitive profile, which has led to the notion of ID as an extremely heterogeneous and variable condition. A genetic syndrome is a disease or disorder that has more than one identifying feature or symptom. Each particular genetic syndrome will have many typical features, depending on which aspects of development are affected by the abnormal genes or chromosomes.

Usually, associated major and minor anomalies (dysmorphic features) are present, accompanied by issues of height/weight growth, psychomotor developmental delay, ID, and behavioural disorders. One of the first studies that showed unusual cognitive profile in children affected by Williams syndrome (WS) was conducted by Thal and colleagues (1989). Subsequently, the group of Bellugi contributed to delineate a typical neuropsychological, neurological, and neuroanatomical profile of WS and Down syndrome (DS), highlighting the relationships between cognition, the brain and, ultimately, the genes involved (Bellugi et al., 1990, 1999; Vicari et al., 2005, 2007; Vicari, 2006). Moreover, in recent years, there has also been much interest around studies of behavioural phenotype in genetic syndromes, in order to identify a relationship between the behavioural aspects of a syndrome and the genotype. A behavioural phenotype, in fact, can be understood as a distinctive pattern in the social, cognitive, and neuropsychological context, associated with a specific genotype (Battaglia & Fisch, 2010). In 1887, John Langdon Down was the first to hypothesize that in the syndrome, later named after him, there were specific personality traits and temperament. The first true description of a "behavioural phenotype" was proposed by William Nyhan in 1971, who described the homonymous syndrome (Lesch Nyhan syndrome) as acts of self-harm, characteristically observed in almost all patients. The importance of defining the cognitive and behavioural phenotype in the context of a syndrome is now widely acknowledged. The current literature covers many descriptions of specific cognitive, psychiatric, and behavioural profiles among the various genetic syndromes, which cannot be explained on the basis of other factors, such as IQ and adaptive functioning. Thus, as for other physical and medical characteristics, such as dysmorphism, heart disease, growth retardation, *etc.*, the definition of the cognitive and behavioural phenotype in genetic syndromes increasingly appears to be a peculiar feature of certain conditions and in a considerable proportion of cases can be considered an important diagnostic tool.

Down and Williams syndrome

DS is a common (though not inherited) genetic disorder caused by an extra copy of chromosome 21 (Lejeune *et al.*, 1959) that affects 1 in 700-800 live births. It is usually associated with a characteristic set of physical features (*e.g.* distinct facial appearance and heart and respiratory problems) and ID, with IQs generally between 35 and 70 (Chapman & Hesketh, 2000). The cognitive profile of people with DS is often characterized by a greater deficit in language than in visuo-spatial abilities. Several studies have revealed a complex neuropsychological profile in this population, with atypical development in both cognitive and linguistic domains (Vicari, 2006). Language is usually compromised since receptive language was found to be stronger than expressive language, and vocabulary to be stronger than syntax (Martin *et al.*, 2009). Broad impairment of the memory domain, particularly verbal short-term memory, is usually documented in individuals with DS. Studies report deficits in verbal and visuo-perceptual long-term memory and relatively spared visuo-spatial long-term memory abilities (Carlesimo *et al.*, 1997; Vicari *et al.*, 2005). These results could be explained by evidence from neuroimaging studies that highlighted anomalies in the hippocampus and medial temporal lobe (Kesslak *et al.*, 1994; Menghini *et al.*, 2011a), as well as a positive correlation of the hippocampus volume with memory measures (Krasuski *et al.*, 2002). Moreover, experimental animal data were generated by a mouse genetic model of DS (Ts65Dn mice) that showed deficits in hippocampus-mediated behavioural tasks and reduced synaptic plasticity of hippocampal pathways (Kleschevnikov *et al.*, 2012). Enhanced efficacy of GABAergic neurotransmission was involved in those changes. It was demonstrated that signalling through postsynaptic GABA(B) receptors is significantly enhanced in the dentate gyrus of Ts65Dn mice. Therefore, Kleschevnikov and collaborators (2012) examined a role for GABA(B) receptors in cognitive deficits in DS by defining the effect of selective GABA(B) receptor antagonists on behaviour and synaptic plasticity in adult Ts65Dn mice. They demonstrated that treatment with the GABA(B) receptor antagonist, CGP55845, improved memory of Ts65Dn mice, in novel place recognition, novel object recognition, and contextual fear conditioning tasks, and increased hippocampal levels of brain-derived neurotrophic factor in the mouse model of DS.

WS is a neurogenetic disorder with an estimated incidence of up to 1 in 7,500 live births (Strømme, 2002), with documented physical, cognitive, behavioural, and neuroanatomical features. It is caused by a hemideletion on chromosome 7q11.23, which includes about 17-25 genes. The medical abnormalities of WS individuals include facial dysmorphism, hyperacusia, and cardiovascular, renal, musculoskeletal, and endocrine malfunctions. Some aspects of language, facial recognition, musical abilities, and social behaviour, with generally "friendly" personality traits, are relatively spared in WS. Instead, spatial, counting, and implicit memory abilities are usually impaired (Mandolesi *et al.*, 2009; Menghini *et al.*, 2010; Vicari *et al.*, 2007). It has been hypothesized that the unique cognitive and behavioural profile of WS could be related to parietal anomalies presented in WS (Menghini *et al.*, 2011b). For example, studies have demonstrated that the corpus callosum of WS individuals shows anomalies in posterior regions since it is shorter, less curved, and significantly thinner compared to controls (Luders *et al.*, 2007). However, in the last few years, specific MRI studies have advanced our understanding of brain anatomy of individuals with genetic syndromes. In particular, a whole-brain unbiased objective technique, known as voxel-based morphometry (VBM), has been developed to characterize brain differences *in vivo* using MRI images. VBM provides an opportunity to assess differences in brain tissue concentrations or volumes between groups (Ashburner & Friston, 2000). Moreover, VBM reduces the risk of investigator bias, because it is minimally operator-dependent and allows the assessment of regional volumetric effects without an *a priori* hypothesis regarding their localization in the brain. In particular, the opportunity to examine all of the voxels representing the cerebrum, the speed with which data is collected and results analyzed compared to manual methods, and the local specificity for grey matter or white matter findings that may be lost in large regional volume manual measures, have led to a gain in popularity for VBM.

The VBM technique has been recently employed for individuals with genetic syndromes and has advanced our understanding of brain anatomy underlying the typical cognitive profile of individuals with ID, particularly, with DS and WS.

Our research group (Menghini *et al.*, 2011a) applied the VMB method using MRI in a group of children and adolescents with DS. To limit differences between brain development, we selected a sample of children with a restricted age range. Twelve children with DS (four girls and eight boys; mean age: 15.5; SD: 2.3 years) and 12 age-matched controls (four girls and eight boys; mean age: 15.6; SD: 2.2) were recruited for the study. Our results documented that, unlike controls, children with DS showed significant local reduction of grey matter density in the left cerebellum, the right hippocampus, the bilateral fusiform gyrus, and the bilateral posterior inferior temporal gyrus. Conversely, they showed a significant increase of grey matter density in the left cerebellar vermis, the left putamen, the left inferior frontal gyrus, the bilateral superior frontal gyrus, and the right posterior superior and middle temporal gyrus. Our data in children with DS confirmed a hippocampal density reduction in this population and a general loss of grey matter density in the medial temporal lobe, probably linked to mnesic and linguistic difficulties, usually observed in individuals with DS. In order to identify structural brain characteristics potentially accounting for specific clinical features of children with DS, we used VBM to directly correlate, with no *a priori* hypothesis for regional changes, brain images and cognitive measures. To this aim, an extensive neuropsychological battery was administered to each child with DS, exploring several cognitive domains, such as global cognitive functioning, linguistic abilities (lexical production and lexical comprehension), sentence repetition and comprehension, phonological and categorical word fluency, visuo-motor and visuo-spatial abilities, and STM abilities (verbal, visual, and spatial short-term memory). Briefly, our correlation results show that a number of brain regions subserve the neuropsychological abilities of participants with DS. Adolescents with DS show typical organization of brain structures related to some cognitive abilities, in particular, spatial memory and visuo-perception (*e.g.* cerebellum and spatial short-term memory; anterior cingulum, medial temporal lobe, and spatial long-term memory; and right middle frontal gyrus and visuo-spatial abilities). However, they present abnormal brain organization related to other cognitive domains, such as linguistic and verbal memory (*e.g.* right middle temporal gyrus and morphosyntactic production; right and left orbitofrontal cortex and verbal long-term memory; and right inferior parietal and verbal short-term memory).

Concerning WS, previous studies have shown inconsistent results when reporting brain abnormalities. This makes the interpretation of clinical and behavioural data challenging in terms of anatomical localization of brain tissue changes. We employed VBM to directly investigate the regional distribution of grey matter density as a function of individual neuropsychological profiles also in individuals with WS. Grey matter maps were regressed against the neuropsychological measures on which WS individuals performed worse than controls. The most consistent finding across VBM studies is the GM reduction in the superior parietal lobe (dorsal stream) of WS individuals (Campbell *et al.*, 2009; Meyer-Lindenberg *et al.*, 2004; Reiss *et al.*, 2004). Our study (Menghini *et al.*, 2011b) confirms this finding, which is claimed to be related to spatial deficits and is considered the most typical neuropsychological feature of WS. The between-group comparisons showed additional regional changes (increased or decreased grey matter density) in individuals with WS. Results also showed an association between the regional grey matter density in the cerebellum, bilaterally, the right supplementary motor area, the right fusiform gyrus, and measures of morpho-syntactic ability. An association was also found between measures of visuo-spatial and visuo-motor abilities and regional grey matter density in the left cerebellum, left parietal lobule, and right superior and left orbital frontal gyri. Reduced grey matter density in these regions might account for, at least partially, some of the visuo-spatial impairments observed in our participants that are typically present in WS. Indeed, it is well known that the posterior parietal and frontal lobes support multimodal spatial representations of body-centred coordinates in humans, as well as in monkeys (Galati *et al.*, 2001). The parietal lobe appears to play a crucial role in producing integrated spatial representations and in planning accurate motor actions. The study shows the potential to clarify the anatomical substrate underlying specific cognitive deficits in WS (Colby & Goldberg, 1999; Rizzolatti *et al.*, 1997). In humans, parietal and frontal lesions may cause a neglect syndrome (Mesulam, 1999). Moreover, neuroimaging studies have shown a role of the parieto-frontal structures in the normal visuo-motor transformations required for reaching and for adaptation to reversed vision (Lacquaniti *et al.*, 1997; Sekiyama *et al.*, 2000). Finally, regarding the relationship between left cerebellum grey matter density and visuo-spatial abilities, previous studies in children with cerebellar lesions have documented the association between left cerebellar damage and visuo-spatial impairment (Riva & Giorgi, 2000).

The controversial findings found in WS individuals are likely related to the abnormalities in their brain shape and size, which introduce a bias during the image pre-processing phase of automated analyses. A further study (Menghini *et al.*, 2013) was conducted to determine whether cerebellar vermis volume measured by the ROI technique differed between a WS sample and a sample of typically developing controls. Although operator-dependent and time-consuming, the ROI is a well-validated approach, it limits bias of automated measures and is strongly indicated especially when there is interest in brain regions with high regional specificity (Menghini *et al.*, 2013). Furthermore, we correlated the vermian volumes with the scores obtained on an extensive neuropsychological battery to identify whether and how cerebellar vermis characteristics are related to specific cognitive features of individuals with WS. This study (Menghini *et al.*, 2013) demonstrated significant volume enlargement of the posterior cerebellar vermis in WS individuals due to an increased volume of lobules VI-VII, as well as atypical width and height ratio of the cerebellar vermis axes. In the light of the enlarged total cerebellar volume in WS, already described in other studies (Campbell *et al.*, 2009; Menghini *et al.*,

2011b), the increased posterior vermis volume appears to be part of a more general pattern of cerebellar enlargement. Although qualitative observations have already documented abnormal cerebellar shape (Schmitt et al., 2001), this is the first study that provides quantitative evidence. The atypical relationship between the width and height of the cerebellar vermis in WS individuals was analyzed using a computer program to directly quantify cerebellar width and height axes. Furthermore, our results documented an inverse correlation between cerebellar vermis volume and scores on some cognitive tasks. In particular, a larger volume of the posterior vermis regions correlated with lower implicit learning, phonological fluency, and verbal short-term memory scores. Our results confirmed findings which extend to the vermis, the well-known contribution in cognition found in lateral cerebellar hemispheres. Moreover, an involvement of cerebellar vermis has been documented in verbal memory, language, and sequence learning (Bolduc et al., 2012; Desmond & Fiez, 1998). Our study furthermore indicated that cerebellar vermis enlargement has a negative effect on the cognitive performance of WS participants. Literature on cerebellar malformation supports the view that cerebellar vermis abnormalities have negative effects on the cognitive profile of a variety of developmental disabilities (Bolduc et al., 2012; Puget et al., 2009; Tavano & Borgatti, 2010).

RAS/MAPK disorders

The RAS/MAPK disorders, defined recently as RASopathies, include Noonan syndrome (NS) and related disorders, such as cardio-facio-cutaneous syndrome, Costello syndrome, LEOPARD syndrome (LS), neurofibromatosis, Noonan-like with loose anagen hair syndrome (recently defined as Mazzanti syndrome), and Legius syndrome (Alfieri et al., 2008). The common denominator of these conditions is the involvement of germinal mutation of genes that encode protein components or modulators of the RAS/MAPK pathway that mediate developmental processes. NS is characterized by postnatal reduced growth, distinctive facial dysmorphism, cardiac defects, and a range of cognitive deficits. Aspects of neurological, visuo-perceptual, and cognitive function in this disorder have been reported in some studies. Motor delay has presumably been attributed to hypotonia, which represents a relatively common feature in affected infants. More significant neurological problems, (e.g. epilepsy) have been noticed in a small minority of individuals. We know that cognitive abilities in NS are often within the normal range, and ID only occurs in approximately 15 per cent of individuals (Cesarini et al., 2009). Heterozygous germline mutations in the *PTPN11*, *SOS1*, *KRAS*, *NRAS*, *RAF1*, *BRAF*, *SHOC2*, and *MEK1* genes account for approximately 75 per cent of individuals with NS (Tartaglia & Gelb, 2010). LS, which phenotypically resembles NS, is characterized by multiple lentigines dispersed throughout the body, *café-au-lait* spots, a higher prevalence of electrocardiographic conduction abnormalities, obstructive cardiomyopathy, and sensorineural hearing deficits. LS and NS are genetically heterogeneous. Mutations in *PTPN11*, *BRAF*, and *RAF1* have been documented to underlie approximately 95 per cent of cases of LS. In animal models, particularly in processes controlling neuronal plasticity, memory, and learning, a crucial role of the RAS/MAPK cascade in cognition has been demonstrated (Sweatt & Weeber, 2003). The activation of the RAS/MAPK pathway has also been observed to be involved in triggering long-term synaptic changes in the mammalian central nervous system (Sweatt & Weeber, 2003), particularly in the hippocampal area CA1 and amygdale, dentate gyrus, and other areas involved in learning and memory (Selcher et al., 2003). Our group conducted various studies in individuals with NS, LS, and other clinically related conditions (*i.e.* cardiofaciocutaneous syndrome and Costello syndrome) associated with different mutations in genes of the RAS/MAPK cascade and indicated that the heterogeneity in cognitive abilities observed in these patients was at least partially attributable to the individual affected genes and type of mutation involved (Cesarini *et al.*, 2009). In particular, mutations in genes that encode transducers, which function upstream of RAS, appear to be less frequently associated with ID since only 12 per cent patients with mutations in *PTPN11* or *SOS1* had low IQ values. In contrast, mutations affecting *HRAS* or genes encoding transducers, which function downstream along the cascade, were more often associated with low IQ scores. In our studies, we found a strong correlation between RASopathies and ID, since in our population only 8 per cent of individuals heterozygous for a *HRAS*, *KRAS*, *RAF1*, *BRAF*, or *MEK1* mutation had an IQ within the normal range. Moreover, our research group evaluated memory and learning in NS and LS and we showed that the profile was not homogeneous across the different domains explored, as long-term memory abilities were lower in the free recall verbal domain while, in visual and spatial recognition domain, long-term memory appeared to be preserved (Alfieri *et al.*, 2011). More specifically, we observed reduced learning in the verbal modality, but relatively little impairment in the visual and spatial modality. These results confirm the crucial role of RAS signalling in memory and learning, as previously demonstrated by experimental animal data generated by murine models that provided evidence for the involvement of RAS/MAPK activation in several tasks of mammalian learning, including fear conditioning, the water maze, and conditioned taste aversion.

Conclusions

In summary, we have reported studies on genetic syndromes demonstrating that genotype influences brain development and cognitive phenotype. The heterogeneity in cognitive abilities and brain neuroanatomy and functioning may be considered to be genetically determined. The individual phenotype encompasses specific cognitive and brain aspects which should be considered to result from specific genes with certain types of mutations.

Conflicts of interest: none.

References

Alfieri, P., Cesarini, L., Zampino, G., *et al.* (2008): Visual function in Noonan and LEOPARD syndrome. *Neuropediatrics* **39**, 335–340.

Alfieri, P., Cesarini, L., Mallardi, M., *et al.* (2011): Long-term memory profile of disorders associated with dysregulation of the RAS-MAPK signaling cascade. *Behav. Genet.* **41**, 423–429.

Ashburner, J. & Friston, K.J. (2000): Voxel-based morphometry-the methods. *Neuroimage* **11**, 805–821.

Battaglia, A. & Fisch, G.S. (2010): Introduction: behavioral phenotypes in neurogenetic syndromes. *Am. J. Med. Genet. C. Semin. Med. Genet.* **154C**, 387–388.

Bellugi, U., Bihrle, A., Jernigan, T., Trauner, D. & Doherty, S. (1990): Neuropsychological, neurological, and neuroanatomical profile of Williams syndrome. *Am. J. Med. Genet. (Suppl)* **6**, 115–125.

Bellugi, U., Lichtenberger, L., Mills, D., Galaburda, A. & Korenberg, J.R. (1999): Bridging cognition, the brain and molecular genetics: evidence from Williams syndrome. *Trends Neurosci.* **22**(5), 197–207.

Bolduc, M.E., du Plessis, A.J., Sullivan, N., *et al.* (2012): Regional cerebellar volumes predict functional outcome in children with cerebellar malformations. *Cerebellum* **11**, 531–542.

Campbell, Z., Zakzanis, K.K., Jovanovski, D., Joordens, S., Mraz, R. & Graham, S.J. (2009): Utilizing virtual reality to improve the ecological validity of clinical neuropsychology: an fMRI case study elucidating the neural basis of planning by comparing the Tower of London with a three-dimensional navigation task. *Appl. Neuropsychol.* **16**, 295–306.

Chapter 13

High-functioning autism spectrum disorders: focus on neuropsychological profiling[1]

Antonio Narzisi*, Filippo Muratori* and Cosimo Urgesi°

*IRCCS Stella Maris Foundation, Dept. of Developmental Neuroscience,
via dei Giacinti 2, 56018 Pisa (Calambrone), Italy;
°University of Udine, Udine, Italy
and IRCCS Scientific Institute 'E. Medea', Pordenone, Italy
antonio.narzisi@fsm.unipi.it, antonionarzisi@yahoo.it, cosimo.urgesi@uniud.it

Summary

Several studies have shown that children with high-functioning autism spectrum disorders are impaired in different cognitive functions, including deficits in motor functions, high-order language aspects, such as semantics and pragmatics, selected executive functions, and memory for faces. On the other hand, there is a growing literature pointing to a relative sparing of visual processing, selected aspects of memory, and inhibitory functions. Results from our studies using NEPSY-II (a unique, co-normed, and multi-domain neuropsychological battery designed specifically for preschoolers, children, and adolescents) showed that only visuo-spatial processing is relatively spared in children with high-functioning autism spectrum disorders, while deficits can be observed in attention and executive functions, language, learning and memory, and sensorimotor processing. Theory of mind difficulties are observed in verbal tasks but not in the understanding of emotional contexts, suggesting that appropriate contextual cues might help emotion understanding in children with high-functioning autism spectrum disorders. These widespread neuropsychological impairments reflect alterations in multiple cognitive domains in high-functioning autism spectrum disorders. Our findings, in particular the lower performances on verbal versus contextual items of theory of mind, may pave the way for empirical studies on larger samples of high-functioning autism spectrum disorders. In conclusion, a detailed investigation of the neuropsychological impairments in high-functioning autism spectrum disorders might help to identify pathophysiological mechanisms associated with the disorder and aid in the design of appropriate interventions aimed at improving cognitive capacities.

Introduction

Individuals with autism spectrum disorders (ASD) exhibit core impairments in the socio-communication domain and have restricted or stereotyped patterns of behaviours. However, ASD vary greatly with regards to the severity of socio-communicative impairments as well as cognitive and language development. ASD with normal or high IQ are referred to as

---

[1] This chapter is a reworking of the manuscript "Neuropsychological profiles in high functioning autism spectrum disorders" published by Narzisi and colleagues (2013) in the *Journal of Autism and Developmental Disorders*.

high-functioning autism (HFA) or high-functioning autism spectrum disorders (HFASD). This term is often used to characterize the broader group of children with HFA, Asperger syndrome, and Pervasive Developmental Disorders Not Otherwise Specified (PDDNOS) (Scheeren et al., 2012). These individuals demonstrate relative strengths in cognitive and language abilities (Klin et al., 2000), though pragmatic language deficits are observed (Landa, 2000). Thus, they share the two core features of ASD: social-communication impairment and circumscribed pattern of behaviour and interest, which, together, contribute to their poor overall social competence (Attwood, 2004).

Several studies have shown that children with HFASD are also impaired in other different cognitive functions (Tsatsanis, 2005), including deficits in motor functions (Baranek et al., 2005), high-order language aspects, such as semantics and pragmatics (Tager-Flusberg, 2004), selected executive functions (Ozonoff et al., 2004), and memory for faces (Hauck et al., 1998). On the other hand, there is a growing literature pointing to a relative sparing of visual processing (Samson et al., 2012), although this is an area of debate (see Edgin & Pennington, 2005), selected aspects of memory (Minshew & Goldstein, 2001), and inhibitory functions (Ozonoff & Strayer, 1997). These findings have contributed to a better knowledge of the cognitive characteristics of HFASD, however, the conclusions that can be drawn from these studies are limited because different tests were used to measure single abilities or a subset of cognitive abilities in different samples of HFASD and control individuals.

NEPSY-II for neuropsychological profiling: review of the topic

The NEPSY is a unique, co-normed, and multi-domain neuropsychological battery designed specifically for preschoolers, children, and adolescents. Its revised version, the NEPSY-II (Korkman et al., 2007), includes measures of social perception abilities, thus also allowing the evaluation of the core deficits of ASD children in comparison to their functioning in other cognitive domains.

In 2013, we conducted a research project aimed at providing a comprehensive description of the neuropsychological profile of children with HFASD (N: 22; mean age: 9.77 years; SD: 3.65; TIQ: 99.09; VIQ: 96.14; PIQ: 103.36) using the NEPSY-II, in order to explore the possible relationships between impairments in different cognitive domains (Urgesi et al., 2011; Narzisi et al., 2013). In keeping with previous studies (Korkman et al., 1998, 2007; Hooper et al., 2006), we expected to find impaired performance for HFASD children in multiple cognitive domains, with particular deficits in attention and executive functions and language and social perception abilities. Importantly, taking into account the mutual influence between executive and language impairments, we tested whether or not the executive deficits in HFASD are secondary to primary deficits in the ability to use inner speech to control and guide behaviours (Hughes & Russell, 1993). Indeed, in keeping with the so-called language mediation hypothesis (Russell et al., 1999), the deficits of HFASD children in executive functions should not be consistent when the relative impact of deficits in language abilities is partialled out.

Neuropsychological profiles of HFASD: NEPSY-II in action

The main aim of our research project was to describe the neuropsychological profiles of HFASD children across different cognitive domains, ruling out the effects of general cognitive abilities. By controlling for verbal general cognitive abilities, several impairments were observed across different cognitive domains in HFASD.

With regards to the attention and executive functioning domain, we confirmed the deficits of HFASD children based on the measures of Inhibition, Animal Sorting and Auditory Attention and Response Set. Furthermore, the pattern of attention and executive function deficits in HFASD was largely consistent with prior research in HFASD using the first version of the NEPSY (Joseph et al., 2005; Hooper et al., 2006; Korkman et al., 1998).

Several studies, indeed, have demonstrated that HFASD children present executive dysfunctions when compared to age-matched typical developing individuals and other clinical control groups (Sergeant et al., 2002; Geurts et al., 2004; Verte et al., 2005). In a similar vein, in other studies that evaluated planning abilities (Ozonoff et al., 2004; Pennington & Ozonoff, 1996; Robinson et al., 2009; Joseph et al., 2005; Happé et al., 2006), HFASD were impaired relative to healthy controls (HC). The NEPSY subtest "Statue" was also used to study two components of motor control: motor response inhibition and motor persistence in 24 patients with HFASD aged 7-13 years (Mahone et al., 2006). Patients with HFASD only achieved lower scores than controls for measures of motor persistence, with no concomitant impairment based on motor inhibition tasks, in keeping with prior research demonstrating relatively spared motor inhibition in autism.

We also confirm the lower performances of HFASD children with respect to the language domain (Hooper et al., 2006; Korkman et al., 2007). In particular, the impairments in phonological processing, oromotor sequences, and repetition of non-sense words are consistent with Tager-Flusberg (2004), who suggested that children with autism and phonological deficits may represent a selected subtype of autism. Whitehouse and collaborators (2008) suggested that only some children with autism demonstrate poor non-sense word repetition, while Schmidt and colleagues (2008) pointed out that problems in phonological processing and repetition of non-sense words might be characteristic of the broad autism phenotype. Accordingly, some studies have found that patients with HFASD have an impairment in the repetition of non-sense words, compared to controls (Riches et al., 2011), and this deficit might reflect a general phonological processing impairment in HFASD (Hooper et al., 2006).

Patients with HFASD had lower performance than HC also in all tasks for the memory and learning domain. These results are consistent with the findings of Korkman and collaborators (2007) and other studies showing impaired immediate memory performance in HFASD. In particular, we confirm that HFASD performance in immediate verbal recall of complex material, such as stories or sentences, is significantly impaired (Minshew & Goldstein, 2001; Williams et al., 2005, 2006). Previous studies have found that individuals with HFASD may display a similar pattern of list learning when the same list of words is repeated five times and presented in the same order (Bowler et al., 2009). However, the impairments of HFASD individuals in verbal learning become particularly apparent under conditions that require organization of the learning material in order to improve performance (Bowler et al., 2010). Such organization of the information is also required by the List Memory and Word List interference tests of the NEPSY-II, in which an interferential list is presented and participants are required to organize the words correctly into two lists, avoiding interference. Thus, the deficits observed in list learning in our HFASD sample may be due mainly to difficulties in organizing the verbal materials and resisting interference, rather than to word learning *per se*. Our results are also consistent with previous evidence, that performance in the immediate recall of complex designs or forms is impaired in ASD children (Minshew & Goldstein, 2001; Williams et al., 2006). We also confirmed the marked deficits in face memory which has been widely reported in the literature. Several studies, indeed, found that patients with ASD, compared to IQ-matched controls, are particularly impaired in this task (Korkman et al., 1998; Klin et al., 1999; Williams *et al.*, 2005; Hooper *et al.*, 2006). However, based on our study, the visuo-spatial memory impairments in HFASD are not limited to faces, but extend to abstract geometric forms (Memory for Designs).

According to Hooper and colleagues (2006), patients with ASD demonstrated deficits in the sensorimotor functions domain. In particular, while no difference between HFASD and control children was observed in the Visuomotor Precision and Finger Tapping tests, specific impairments were found in the imitation of hand postures and in the manual motor sequences tests, *i.e.* in those tasks requiring the imitation of complex movement sequences. Following Joseph and collaborators (2005), these tasks require children to combine working memory and inhibitory control in order to withhold a dominant motor response by maintaining a conflicting response rule (*e.g.* to knock with one hand while the other hand taps, and vice versa) in active memory. In keeping with our finding, Korkman and colleagues (2007) and Hooper and collaborators (2006) showed no significant differences between HFASD versus controls in the Finger Tapping task, suggesting the absence of deficits in low-level sensorimotor control.

The findings regarding the social perception domain confirm the results of Korkman and colleagues (2007) with lower scores for HFASD than controls in Affect Recognition and Theory of Mind Verbal tasks. Concerning the social perception domain, an important result of our study was the intact performances of HFASD in the contextual items of the Theory of Mind test.

These trials evaluate the capacity of children to understand how certain emotions are linked to given social situations and to recognize correctly the emotions that the various social settings generate. The child is shown an illustration of a social situation and he/she has to choose which of four facial expressions illustrates appropriately the emotional state of one of the characters shown in the photograph. Our results contrast with those of Da Fonseca and collaborators (2008) which revealed that children with HFASD are able to use contextual cues to recognize objects, but not emotions. However, in contrast to the task of Da Fonseca and colleagues (2008), in which the children had to choose the appropriate emotional state between smile illustrations, in the NEPSY-II tasks, the children had to choose the appropriate emotional state from photographs of real faces. Our findings may suggest that: (1) contextual elements (the social situation) appear to facilitate the processing of the corresponding emotional state (photograph of a human face); (2) the human face, in contrast to illustrations of smiling (Da Fonseca *et al.*, 2008), could facilitate the activation of an isomorphic process (the identity between the level of observed experience and that of the physiological processes underlying it) in HFASD children (Eagle & Wakefield, 2007; Gallese, 2003); (3) the systematizing inclination of HFASD to analyze details (Baron-Cohen, 2010) could facilitate the trend toward greater attention to contextual cues of social situations by facilitating the recognition of appropriate emotional states.

Our HFASD sample displayed a relative sparing of visuo-spatial abilities when compared with the severe neuropsychological deficits observed in the other domains. In this domain, only the Arrows and Design Copy tests showed a significant difference between the HFASD and HC children, with scores corresponding to borderline performance. The deficits in line orientation discrimination (the Arrows test) have also been found in previous studies (Korkman *et al.*, 2007; Hooper *et al.*, 2006). On the other hand, the deficit in the Design Copying test is consistent with the initial validation study of the NEPSY-II (Korkman *et al.*, 2007), but not with the validation study of the NEPSY (Hooper *et al.*, 2006). This discrepancy between the two tests might be due to the improvement of the sensitivity of the Design Copy test in the NEPSY-II, with the inclusion of more complex items. Importantly, only the motor and global processing scores of the Design Copying test were lower in HFASD than HC children, while no difference was found in the local processing score. Thus, while HFASD children presented difficulties in fine-motor control, causing inaccurate drawing and representation of the overall configuration of the design, they accurately represented the design features. This suggests a bias of HFASD children towards a local strategy of stimulus processing (Baron-Cohen, 2010), which may be detected by analyzing the specific processing scores of the NEPSY-II Design Copying test.

Conclusion

In conclusion, our study supports the utility of NEPSY-II as a sensitive evaluation tool to describe the neuropsychological profile of HFASD children. It can identify weaknesses and strengths of their cognitive abilities, and distinguish between primary and secondary deficits. Furthermore, our findings, in particular the lower performances on verbal versus contextual items of Theory of Mind, may pave the way for empirical studies on larger samples of HFASD. Indeed, a detailed investigation of the neuropsychological impairments in HFASD might help to identify the pathophysiological mechanisms associated with the disorder and aid in the design of appropriate interventions aimed at improving cognitive capacities.

Conflicts of interest: none.

References

Attwood, T. (2004): Cognitive behaviour therapy for children and adults with Asperger's syndrome. *Behav. Change* **21**, 147–162.

Baranek, G., Parham, L.D. & Bodfish, J.W. (2005): Sensory and motor features in autism: assessment and intervention. In: *Handbook of Autism and Pervasive Developmental Disorders*, eds. F.R. Volkmar, R. Paul, A. Klin, & D. Cohen, vol. 2. New York: John Wiley & Sons.

Baron-Cohen, S. (2010): Empathizing, systemizing, and the extreme male brain theory of autism. *Prog. Brain Res.* **186**, 167–175.

Bowler, D.M., Limoges, E. & Mottron, L. (2009): Different verbal learning strategies in autism spectrum disorder: evidence from the Rey Auditory Verbal Learning Test. *J. Aut. Dev. Disord.* **39**, 910–915.

Bowler, D.M., Gaigg, S.B. & Gardiner, J.M. (2010): Multiple list learning in adults with autism spectrum disorder: parallels with frontal lobe damage or further evidence of diminished relational processing? *J. Aut. Dev. Disord.* **40**, 179–187.

Da Fonseca, D., Santos, A., Bastard-Rosset, D., Rondan, C., Poinso, F. & Deruelle, C. (2008): Can children with autistic spectrum disorders extract emotions out of contextual cues? *Res. Aut. Spect. Disord.* **3**, 50–56.

Eagle, M.N. & Wakefield, J.M. (2007): Gestalt psychology and the mirror neuron discovery. *Gestalt Theory* **29**, 54–64.

Edgin, J.O. & Pennington B.F. (2005): Spatial cognition in autism spectrum disorders: superior, impaired, or just intact? *J. Aut. Dev. Disord.* **35**, 729–745.

Gallese, V. (2003): The manifold nature of interpersonal relations: the quest for a common mechanism. *Philosophical Transactions of the Royal Society of London. Series B, Biological Sciences* **358**, 517–528.

Geurts, H.M., Verté, S., Oosterlaan, J., Roeyers, H. & Sergeant, J.A. (2004). How specific are executive functioning deficits in attention deficit hyperactivity disorder and autism? *J. Child Psychol. Psychiatry* **45**, 836–854.

Happé, F., Booth, R., Charlton, R. & Hughes C. (2006): Executive function deficits in autism spectrum disorders and attention-deficit/hyperactivity disorder: examining profiles across domains and ages. *Brain Cogn.* **61**, 25–39.

Hauck, M., Fein, D., Maltby, N., Waterhouse, L. & Feinstein, C. (1998): Memory for faces in children with autism. *Child Neuropsychol.* **4**, 187–198.

Hooper, S.R., Poon, K.K., Marcus, L. & Fine, C. (2006): Neuropsychological characteristics of school-age children with high-functioning autism: performance on the NEPSY. *Child Neuropsychol.* **12**, 299–305.

Joseph, R.M., McGrath, L.M. & Tager-Flusberg, H. (2005): Executive dysfunction and its relation to language ability in verbal school-age children with autism. *Dev. Neuropsychol.* **27**, 361–378.

Chapter 14

Cognitive and language development in children with early focal brain lesions

Anna Maria Chilosi, Paola Brovedani, Sara Lenzi, Paola Cristofani and Paola Cipriani

*Dept. of Developmental Neuroscience, IRCCS Stella Maris,
viale del Tirreno 331, 56128 Calambrone, Pisa, Italy*
achilosi@fsm.unipi.it

Summary

Plasticity of the developing brain after early focal brain lesions (EFBL) has been largely demonstrated by a bulk of research documenting the high potential for post-lesional reorganization of the neural substrate and of linguistic and cognitive functions. Several studies reveal that cognitive function is relatively preserved in children with EFBL, particularly for verbal rather than performance skills. Even if cognitive outcome is not easily predictable, some factors (*e.g.* the presence of epilepsy) may negatively affect cognitive development and may be associated with a worse cognitive outcome. The decline of cognitive performance reported in some studies may not necessarily reflect a loss of skills, but rather a slower gain over time and difficulties with increasing task demands. With regards to language development, it has been shown that children with early brain injuries, involving the classic language areas of the left hemisphere, are able to learn the basic rules of oral language, although they may show some difficulties in the acquisition of more complex and later emerging verbal abilities. Moreover, the few available studies show that a significant proportion of children with EFBL and normal cognitive development also have difficulties in the acquisition of academic skills with a greater incidence of specific learning disorders, in comparison to healthy children.

Introduction

The study of early focal brain lesions (EFBL) provides a unique opportunity to investigate the relationship between cognitive and language functions and their cerebral substrates, in a condition in which early damage may force brain plasticity to organize linguistic and other cognitive abilities into alternative circuitries. Early lesions impact developing distributed functional networks that sustain cognitive abilities, which are characterized by progressive specialization and localization of function. The adult domain-specific modularization may be the end state of development. The association between structure and function changes during development, with the same behaviours supported by different neural substrates at different ages (Johnson, 2011; Power *et al.*, 2010).

The effects of congenital non-progressive focal brain lesions on behavioural outcome depend on lesion type, localization, and extension, and the age at which they arise. Brain lesions occurring at the beginning of the third trimester of gestation are generally due to periventricular venous infarction that leads to periventricular leukomalacia (PVL), whereas cortical and subcortical grey matter lesions are generally associated with injuries occurring towards the end of the third trimester. Not all infants with early brain injury will develop neurocognitive, postural and movement deficits (hemiplegia, diplegia, tetraplegia). Neurocognitive outcome may depend on different lesion factors as well as other variables, such as the presence of epilepsy, cerebral visual impairment, and premature birth. Identifying which children may develop negative cognitive and behavioural sequelae as a consequence of early lesions is a current and very challenging topic of investigation.

Cognitive development after unilateral early focal brain lesions

Cognitive outcome of children with EFBL is still controversial, despite the large amount of published reports on this topic and early prediction of cognitive development still remains a challenge (*e.g.* Van Buuren *et al.*, 2013). Across studies, the variability in intelligent quotients (IQs), or Developmental Quotients (DQs), is largely due to differences in inclusion criteria (*e.g.* children with/without cerebral palsy; with/without other associated impairments such as visual deficits or epilepsy) and in the analysis of lesion characteristics that need to be carefully defined in order to allow more accurate predictions on cognitive status (*e.g.* Ballantyne *et al.*, 2008; Ricci *et al.*, 2008; Riva *et al.*, 2012). Several authors have reported cognitive skills in the normal-low average range in most children, both after white matter lesions (PVL) and cortical damage (Ballantyne *et al.*, 2007; Chilosi *et al.*, 2001; Ricci *et al.*, 2008; Riva *et al.*, 2012; Westmacott *et al.*, 2010) with no significant effect of the side of lesion on Verbal IQ (VIQ) or Performance IQ (PIQ). The presence of seizures, but also of EEG abnormalities, has a detrimental effect on intelligence (Gonzalez-Monge *et al.*, 2009; Riva *et al.*, 2012; Vargha-Khadem *et al.*, 1992). There have been relatively few longitudinal studies on the stability of intellectual development over time and the results on long-term outcome are often conflicting.

A relatively stable pattern of intellectual performance was already reported in earlier studies by Aram and Eisele (1994) and has more recently been confirmed by Ballantyne and colleagues (2008) and Gonzalez-Monge and collaborators (2009) with a sparing of VIQ with respect to PIQ, which instead decreases in time. Cognitive stability indicates that the brain is able to compensate after early injury and may maintain a steady rate of development, albeit at a lower level than that of normal controls. However, stability may not be evident early on in development after congenital unilateral focal brain lesions.

In the longitudinal study of Chilosi and co-workers (2001) on early cognitive and language development of hemiplegic children with congenital focal brain lesions (documented at MRI), a slowing down of cognitive performances was observed between the second and fourth year of life. In this study, 18 children, nine with left and nine with right hemisphere damage (LHD and RHD), where evaluated with the Griffiths Mental Developmental Scales at about 2 (Time 1) and 4 years of age (Time 2). At the first observation period (mean age: 23 months), cognitive profiles across subscales showed side-specific effects resembling the adult left/right cerebral hemisphere lesion model. Not only did LHD children score significantly lower than RHD on the Hearing and Speech subscale, but they presented higher Performance than Hearing and Speech quotients. Conversely, the RHD group had higher Hearing and Speech than Performance developmental quotients. The above patterns appeared to hold over time, but damage to either hemisphere was associated with a slowing down of the rate of development between Time 1 and Time 2. Indeed, at the second observation (mean age: 38 months), a decrement of cognitive efficiency emerged, as documented by a lowering of the mean Global Developmental quotient.

Other longitudinal studies have found evidence of cognitive decline during school age (Levine *et al.*, 2005; Van Buuren *et al.*, 2013; Westmacott *et al.*, 2010). Van Buuren and co-workers have recently analyed cognitive outcome at school age of 50 children with unilateral brain lesions due to periventricular haemorrhagic infarction (21 subjects; 57 per cent with unilateral spastic cerebral palsy) and perinatal arterial ischaemic stroke (29 subjects; 48 per cent with hemiplegia). Cognitive assessment was performed at a median age of 24 months (range: 18-32 months) by means of the Griffiths Mental Developmental Scales and at a mean age of 11 years and 9 months (range: 6-20 years) by means of the Wechsler Scales. Cognitive abilities at school age were below average, but still within one standard deviation from the mean for most children. According to the authors, prediction of cognitive outcome remains challenging, but some early predictors can be hypothesized. In the case of periventricular haemorrhagic infarction, cognitive scores fell outside the normal range in infancy, but there was no further decline at school age. Cognitive outcome of children with perinatal arterial ischaemic stroke was more variable, and 16 of 29 children showed a significant decline in intellectual ability over time. Involvement of basal ganglia and thalami and the presence of post-neonatal epilepsy were associated with worse cognitive outcome. According to the authors, the role of thalamic injury in regulating information transmission to the cortex and among cortical areas may be critical in determining lower cognitive skills and its involvement represents a risk factor for cognitive outcome.

Concerning the effects of lesion side on outcome, sparing of verbal abilities with respect to performance skills, irrespective of lesion laterality, has been reported, suggesting language priority for human development that has been referred to as "verbal sparing" (Ballantyne *et al.*, 2008; Gonzalez-Monge *et al.*, 2009; Nass *et al.*, 1992; Riva & Cazzaniga, 1986; Riva *et al.*, 2012). In the case of right hemisphere lesions, visuo-spatial abilities may be selectively impaired, as demonstrated by studies, albeit few in number, addressing non-verbal functions (Kolk & Talvik, 2000; Lidzba *et al.*, 2006a, 2006b; Stiles-Davis *et al.*, 1988).

In an ongoing study of a group of hemiplegic children with Full Scale IQ (FSIQ) greater than 80 (21 with LHD and 11 with RHD; mean age: 10 years and 6 months), longitudinally evaluated at the Scientific Institute Stella Maris (Chilosi *et al.*, in preparation), VIQ, PIQ and FSIQ did not differ as a function of lesion side. The majority of children had higher VIQ than PIQ, although the difference was not statistically significant.

Altogether, these data indicate that, in the case of pre-perinatal focal brain lesions, cognitive skills are not severely impaired, but cognitive outcome is not easily predictable. It is worth noting that the decline of cognitive performance reported in some studies may not necessarily reflect a loss of skills, but rather a slower gain over time and difficulties with increasing task demands and higher cognitive requirements that may not be adequate in comparison with healthy peers.

Language development in children with unilateral early focal brain lesions

A series of cross-sectional and longitudinal studies on the early phases of language acquisition of children with pre-perinatal brain damage revealed delayed achievement of early developmental milestones, including late onset of babbling and first words in patients with both left and right hemisphere lesions.

In a series of seminal studies by Bates and her colleagues on early language acquisition after unilateral congenital lesions (not necessarily associated with hemiplegia) (Bates et al., 1992, 1997; Thal et al., 1991; Vicari et al., 2000), the effects of both the stage of language development and the site/side of injury were specifically addressed.

The study by Thal and co-workers (1991) on RHD and LHD children showed that in the period from 10 to 17 months of age, both groups presented a delay in language production, with RHD children being at greater risk of delay in word comprehension and gestures than LHD children. The subsequent study by Bates and colleagues (1997) confirmed these results on a larger sample, specifying that in the first two years of life, children with LHD had a selective delay in lexical production, whereas children with RHD had a greater delay in the production of communicative and symbolic gestures. In the period from 10 to 44 months, the delay was maintained, especially in lexicon and grammar (Vicari et al., 2000). In particular, a significantly greater delay in expressive vocabulary and grammar was associated with a lesion involving the left temporal lobe. However, in contrast to adults with focal left temporal injuries (who show fluent aphasia, often accompanied by moderate-to-severe deficits in comprehension), none of the children with left temporal injury had a receptive language deficit in addition to the expressive delay.

Prospective studies by Chilosi and co-workers (2001, 2005) on individual trajectories of language acquisition in hemiplegic RHD and LHD children, assessed around the second and fourth year of life, confirmed the initial delay in speech and language development irrespective of lesion side, although, in LHD, the delay in expressive vocabulary and grammar was more marked. With increasing age, both groups increased vocabulary size and grammar, but language production was still lagging behind, compared to normal peers, more often in LHD than RHD children.

In general, the above studies show that children with unilateral EFBL do not manifest true aphasic symptoms and effects due to both lesion side and site are no longer detectable after 7 years of age, documenting a considerable recovery after the early pre-school years (Bates & Roe, 2001; Reilly et al., 1998, 2004).

In a cross-sectional study on narrative abilities of children aged 3 to 10 years, Reilly and collaborators (1998) found positive changes with age in lexical production and morphological, syntactic, and narrative complexity. However, it was reported that, in contrast to peers with normal development, it was only at around 8-10 years of age that children with either right or left hemisphere injury performed in the normal range with regards to morphology, use of complex syntax, and narrative structure (Reilly et al., 1998, 2004). Interestingly, in the youngest group (ages 4 to 6), LHD children made more morphosyntactic errors than RHD and control subjects, but from age seven onwards, there were no side or site-specific effects (Reilly et al., 1998). Similar results were reported by Demir and co-workers (2010) who found, in a group of 11 children with unilateral EFBL aged 5 to 8 years, oral language difficulties on a variety of measures including narrative length, diversity of vocabulary, and narrative structure.

In general, school-aged children with LHD or RHD go on to attain good functional language abilities in free speech situations and can use language in the context of everyday communication without marked impairment. They are able to learn basic grammar rules and do not show morphological deficits. In the study of Marchman and colleagues (2004), children with unilateral EFBL (mean age: 6.5 years) were not more likely, relative to children with normal development, to produce past tense errors, which have been considered hallmark signs of Specific Language Impairment (SLI), and no significant differences in error scores were observed in relation to the side of lesion.

However, some studies on the acquisition of complex language at school age have shown that difficulties may reappear when children are faced with new linguistic challenges, as demonstrated by low scores in complex narrative tasks. Discourse expression difficulties were reported by Chapman and co-workers (2003) in a study on adolescents who suffered from unilateral stroke occurring in the perinatal period.

Reilly and co-workers (2013), in a study on later language and discourse skills in children with perinatal stroke (ages 7 to 16 years), found that they could meet age-appropriate daily conversational demands, but creating and organizing a narrative, especially an emotionally salient one, was a challenging task for them. Moreover, LHD subjects made more morphological errors and used less complex syntax and fewer syntactic types than controls; they also produced impoverished story settings. In contrast, RHD subjects performed comparably to controls, except for scarce use of complex syntax.

Below-average performance, based on an extensive battery of language tests (Clinical Evaluation of Language Function [CELF-R]; Semel *et al.*, 1987), was reported by Ballantyne and co-workers (2007) who studied a group of 28 children with perinatal unilateral ischaemic stroke, 62 per cent of whom had hemiplegia. The subjects (aged 7 to 16) scored significantly below the norm in both production and comprehension, independent of lesion side. Clinical and neuroanatomical characteristics of the lesion, such as laterality of focal seizure and site or severity of injury, were not linearly associated with language outcome and in most cases were not predictive of language performance. Over a 3-year period, there was no regression in performance, rather, a stability in language functioning. A history of seizures was associated with a further decrease in scores on language tests (Ballantyne *et al.*, 2008).

The studies summarized above reveal that left hemisphere lesions do not undermine the ability to learn language, even when damage involves the classic adult language areas, although the level of complex verbal skills may be below that of age-matched controls.

The effects of unilateral early local brain lesions on cerebral lateralization and specialization

Concerning the effects of pre-perinatal brain lesions on cerebral lateralization and specialization, neuropsychological studies provided evidence that, in the case of left congenital lesions, the reallocation of verbal functions to the right hemisphere may lead to a reorganization of the neural substrate and cognitive functions. Atypical hemispheric lateralization for language, in terms of a shift of language processing to the right hemisphere, has been demonstrated by several studies that used the dichotic listening test (Brizzolara *et al.*, 2002; Carlsson *et al.*, 1992; Chilosi *et al.*, 2005; Isaacs *et al.*, 1996) and confirmed by functional MRI (fMRI) data (*e.g.* Guzzetta *et al.*, 2008). In a study by Chilosi and co-workers (2005) with a fused dichotic listening paradigm, an atypical lateralization for language was found in a high percentage of LHD children and it was strongly associated with delayed language development. Atypical lateralization coefficients were also present in some RHD children, suggesting that early unilateral brain damage to either hemisphere alters normal lateralization patterns, probably reducing the contribution of the damaged hemisphere and enhancing that of the intact one in language processing.

In a collaborative study with Daria Riva's research group at the Fondazione IRCCS Istituto Neurologico 'C. Besta' (Milan), supported by the Mariani Foundation (project title: Validation of neurofunctional and behavioural techniques for the assessment of language lateralization and development in exceptional circumstances: children with early focal brain lesions and children with cochlear implants), functional transcranial doppler ultrasound (fTCD) and fMRI were used to investigate language lateralization in children with early left focal brain lesions and age- and sex-matched normal controls. fTCD uses ultrasounds to measure event-related changes in blood flow in the middle cerebral arteries and it may be used to evaluate cerebral activation during various linguistic tasks (Bishop et al., 2009).

Our research demonstrated that fTCD is a sensitive measure of cerebral dominance for language during development and correlates well with fMRI data. It was well tolerated by all children, confirming its potential use as a clinical tool, particularly suitable for the evaluation of hemispheric lateralization in young children (a critical factor in terms of its clinical usability).

Our study is the first to compare the hemispheric lateralization indexes (LIs) obtained with fTCD and fMRI, in patients with early focal brain lesions. In accordance with a large body of literature, in normal controls, LIs obtained with the two methods indicated a dominance of the left hemisphere for language in the majority of individuals. In particular, the proportion of left-hemisphere-dominant subjects was above 84 per cent in the case of both fTCD and fMRI.

The pattern of lateralization of subjects with LHD was reversed with respect to normal controls because of a shift of cerebral dominance for language in a high proportion of individuals. This finding is in keeping with previous studies carried out with fMRI. In particular, in the study by Guzzetta and colleagues (2008), ten children with left perinatal arterial stroke, right hemiplegia, and normal cognitive functions were administered a covert rhyme generation task. Eight showed a right-hemisphere lateralization for language, including all five patients with a damaged left Broca's area and three without involvement of Broca's area. Group analysis of patients with right hemispheric language organisation showed brain activations homotopic to those found in the left hemisphere of a matched control group. These findings are in agreement with the results of other functional imaging studies reporting right hemisphere processing of language stimuli after perinatal periventricular white matter lesions (Staudt et al., 2001) and after left hemisphere stroke (Tillema et al., 2008).

The shift of language to the right hemisphere may not determine significant language deficits because of the capacity of the right hemisphere to compensate early damage (Satz et al., 1994; Teuber, 1975). Nevertheless, according to Teuber's hypothesis (1975), reorganization of language processing in the right hemisphere may occur at the expense of non-verbal visual spatial functions subsumed by this hemisphere. This "cost" in terms of plasticity has been referred to by Teuber as a "crowding effect" and has been documented by studies showing higher verbal than performance quotients both in children with right and left lesions (Ballantyne et al., 2008; Gonzalez-Monge et al., 2009; Nass et al., 1992; Riva & Cazzaniga, 1986; Riva et al., 2012).

Direct evidence supporting the crowding hypothesis has been provided by two fMRI studies conducted by Lidzba and co-workers (Lidzba et al., 2006a, 2006b) on adults with right hemiplegia due to left-hemisphere perinatal lesions (unilateral periventricular or cortical-subcortical damage). In the first study (Lidzba et al., 2006a), patients who had right hemisphere activation for language on fMRI presented visuo-spatial deficits which were absent in patients with lesions on the left side, in whom the right hemisphere was not activated. Moreover, the degree of right hemisphere involvement in language processing was correlated with the degree of visuo-spatial deficit. In the second study (Lidzba et al., 2006b), the authors reported that in patients with right-hemisphere language organization, verbal and non-verbal functions shared the same right hemisphere network. Moreover, the lesion (independently of size) seemed to prevent compensatory use of the left hemisphere.

According to the authors: "the functional disadvantage of the originally right hemisphere network might be explained by the fact that complex visuo-spatial skills develop later in childhood (Fine *et al.*, 2003) than language, which has reached a rather complex level already at the age of three".

Acquisition of academic skills in EFBL children

In the literature, very few studies have analyzed the incidence of specific learning difficulties in EFBL children with normal intelligence. The available studies have documented a greater incidence of specific difficulties in written language and mathematics in children with hemiplegia and normal cognitive development, compared to healthy children (Anderson *et al.*, 2009; Ballatyne *et al.*, 2008; Frampton *et al.*, 1998; Frith & Vargha-Khadem, 2001). In the study of Frampton and co-workers (Frampton *et al.*, 1998), more than one third of the 59 hemiplegic children (35.6 per cent), equally represented by children with LHD and RHD, presented specific learning difficulties in at least one domain (writing, reading, and arithmetical skills) and around half had deficits in two or more domains despite average IQ. Frith and Vargha-Khadem (2001), based on a heterogeneous group of children with hemiplegia (38 with perinatal and 15 with postnatal injury), found that left hemisphere injury in males was more detrimental for reading and spelling than right-sided damage. Performance of females with either left or right-sided damage was age-appropriate.

In our ongoing study (Chilosi *et al.*, in preparation), about one third of 32 hemiplegic children (mean age: 10.6; range: 7-18; 21 with LHD and 11 with RHD) presented specific reading disabilities. Reading performance did not differ between LHD and RHD subjects and was not correlated with either lesion type (stroke or periventricular damage) or number of lobes involved.

Moreover, reading decoding skills did not correlate with cognitive abilities, whereas text comprehension significantly correlated with WISC-III or WAIS-R Full Scale and Verbal IQ (FSIQ $p = .002$; VIQ $p = .001$).

These data document the long-term effects of early brain lesions and how they may influence not only early, but also later stages of oral and written language acquisition.

Conclusion

The literature on neuropsychological profiles of subjects with EFBL shows the extraordinary plasticity of the developing brain that is able to recover many functions after cerebral damage. In contrast to acquired lesions in the adult, congenital left hemisphere damage does not determine aphasic symptoms, even when it involves the classic language areas. The neurofunctional reorganization, however, has some short and long-term costs in terms of intellectual abilities, complex language acquisition, and academic achievements. These long-lasting effects are mainly independent of the side of lesion, but may be influenced by factors such as presence of epilepsy and lesion type.

New methods for exploring the child's brain may contribute to a better understanding of the mechanisms underlying functional reorganization and environmental effects (early remediation and training of specific cognitive functions).

Conflicts of interest: none.

References

Anderson, V., Spencer-Smith, M., Leventer, R., et al. (2009): Childhood brain insult: can age at insult help us predict outcome? *Brain* **132,** 45–56.

Aram, D.M. & Eisele, J.A. (1994): Intellectual stability in children with unilateral brain lesions. *Neuropsychologia* **32,** 85–95.

Ballantyne, A.O., Spilkin, A.M. & Trauner, D.A. (2007): Language outcome after perinatal stroke: does side matter? *Child Neuropsychol.* **13,** 494–509.

Ballantyne, A.O., Spilkin, A.M., Hesselink, J. & Trauner, D.A. (2008): Plasticity in the developing brain: intellectual, language and academic functions in children with ischaemic perinatal stroke. *Brain* **131,** 2975–2985.

Bates, E. & Roe, K. (2001): Language development in children with unilateral brain injury. In: *Handbook of Developmental Cognitive Neuroscience,* eds. C.A. Nelson & M. Luciana. Cambridge, MA: MIT Press, pp. 281–307.

Bates, E., Thal, D. & Janowsky, J.S. (1992): Early language development and its neural correlates. In: *Handbook of Neuropsychology,* eds. S.J. Segalowitz & I. Rapin. Amsterdam: Elsevier, pp. 69–110.

Bates, E., Thal, D., Aram, D., Eisele, J., Nass, R. & Trauner, D. (1997): From first words to grammar in children with focal brain injury. *Dev. Neuropsychol.* **13,** 275–343.

Bishop, D.V.M., Watt, H. & Papadatou-Pastou, M. (2009). An efficient and reliable method for measuring cerebral lateralization during speech with functional transcranial Doppler ultrasound. *Neuropsychologia* **47,** 587–590.

Brizzolara, D., Pecini, C., Brovedani, P., Ferretti, G., Cipriani, P. & Cioni, G. (2002): Timing and type of congenital brain lesion determine different patterns of language lateralization in hemiplegic children. *Neuropsychologia* **40,** 620–632.

Carlsson, G., Hugdahl, K., Uvebrant, P., Wiklund, L.M. & von Wendt, L. (1992): Pathological left-handedness revisited: dichotic listening in children with left vs right congenital hemiplegia. *Neuropsychologia* **30,** 471–481.

Chapman, S.B., Max, J.E., Gamino, J.F., McGlothlin, J.H. & Cliff, S.N. (2003): Discourse plasticity in children after stroke: age at injury and lesion effects. *Pediatr. Neurol.* **29,** 34–41.

Chilosi, A.M., Cipriani, P., Bertuccelli, B., Pfanner, L. & Cioni, G. (2001): Early cognitive and communication development in children with focal brain lesions. *J. Child Neurol.* **16,** 309–316.

Chilosi, A.M., Pecini, C., Cipriani, P., et al. (2005): Atypical language lateralization and early linguistic development in children with focal brain lesions. *Dev. Med. Child Neurol.* **47,** 725–730.

Demir, O.E., Levine, S.C. & Goldin-Meadow, S. (2010): Narrative skill in children with early unilateral brain injury: a possible limit to functional plasticity. *Dev. Sci.* **13,** 636–647.

Fine, I., Wade, A.R., Brewer, A.A., et al. (2003): Long-term deprivation affects visual perception and cortex. *Nat. Neurosci.* **6,** 915–916.

Frampton, I., Yude, C. & Goodman, R. (1998): The prevalence and correlates of specific learning difficulties in a representative sample of children with hemiplegia. *Br. J. Educ. Psychol.* **68,** 39–51.

Frith, U. & Vargha-Khadem, F. (2001): Are there sex differences in the brain basis of literacy related skills? Evidence from reading and spelling impairments after early unilateral brain damage. *Neuropsychologia* **39,** 1485–1488.

Gonzalez-Monge, S., Boudia, B., Ritz, A., et al. (2009): A 7-year longitudinal follow-up of intellectual development in children with congenital hemiplegia. *Dev. Med. Child Neurol.* **51,** 959–967.

Guzzetta, A., Pecini, C., Biagi, L., et al. (2008): Language organisation in left perinatal stroke. *Neuropediatrics* **39,** 157–163.

Isaacs, E., Christie, D., Vargha-Kadem, F. & Mishkin, M. (1996): Effects of hemispheric side of injury, age at injury, and presence of seizure disorder on functional ear and hand asymmetries in hemiplegic children. *Neuropsychologia* **34,** 127–137.

Johnson, M.H. (2011): Interactive specialization: a domain-general framework for human functional brain development? *Dev. Cogn. Neurosc.* **1,** 7–21.

Kolk, A. & Talvik, T. (2000): Cognitive outcome of children with early-onset hemiparesis. *J. Child Neurol.* **15,** 581–587.

Levine, S.C., Kraus, R., Alexander, E., Suriyakham L.W. & Huttenlocher, P.R. (2005): IQ decline following early unilateral brain injury: a longitudinal study. *Brain Cogn.* **59,** 114–123.

Lidzba, K., Staudt, M., Wilke, M. & Krägeloh-Mann, I. (2006a): Visuospatial deficits in patients with early left-hemispheric lesions and functional reorganization of language: consequence of lesion or reorganization? *Neuropsychologia* **44,** 1088–1094.

Lidzba, K., Staudt, M., Wilke, M., Grodd, W. & Krägeloh-Mann, I. (2006b): Lesion-induced right-hemispheric language and organization of nonverbal functions. *Neuroreport* **17,** 929–933.

Marchman, V.A., Saccuman, C. & Wulfeck, B. (2004): Productive use of the English past tense in children with focal brain injury and specific language impairment. *Brain Lang.* **88,** 202–214.

Nass, R., Sadler, A.E. & Sidtis, J.J. (1992): Differential effects of congenital versus acquired unilateral brain injury on dichotic listening performance: evidence for sparing and asymmetric crowding. *Neurology* **42,** 1960–1965.

Power, J.D., Fair, D.A., Schlaggar, B.L. & Petersen, S.E. (2010): The development of human functional brain networks. *Neuron* **67**(5), 735–748.

Reilly, J.S., Bates, E.A. & Marchman, V.A. (1998): Narrative discourse in children with early focal brain injury. *Brain Lang.* **61,** 335–375.

Reilly, J., Losh, M., Bellugi, U. & Wulfeck, B. (2004): 'Frog, where are you?' Narratives in children with specific language impairment, early focal brain injury, and Williams syndrome. *Brain Lang.* **88,** 229–247.

Reilly, J.S., Wasserman, S. & Appelbaum, M. (2013): Later language development in narratives in children with perinatal stroke. *Dev. Sci.* **16,** 67–83.

Ricci, D., Mercuri, E., Barnett, A., *et al.* (2008): Cognitive outcome at early school age in term-born children with perinatally acquired middle cerebral artery territory infarction. *Stroke* **39,** 403–410.

Riva, D. & Cazzaniga, L. (1986): Late effects of unilateral brain lesions sustained before and after age one. *Neuropsychologia* **4,** 423–428.

Riva, D., Franceschetti, S., Erbetta, A., Baranello, G., Esposito, S. & Bulgheroni, S. (2012): Congenital brain damage: cognitive development correlates with lesion and electroencephalographic features. *J. Child Neurol.* **28,** 446–454.

Satz, P., Strauss, E., Hunter, M. & Wada, J. (1994): Re-examination of the crowing hypothesis: effects of age of onset. *Neuropsychol.* **8,** 255–262.

Semel, E., Wiig, E.H. & Secord, W. (1987): *Clinical Evaluation of Language Fundamentals-Revised (CELF-R).* San Antonio, TX: PsychCorp, Pearson.

Staudt, M., Grodd, W., Niemann, G., Wildgruber, D., Erb, M. & Krägeloh-Mann, I. (2001): Early left periventricular brain lesions induce right hemispheric organization of speech. *Neurology* **57**(1): 122–125.

Stiles-Davis, J., Janowsky, J., Engel, M. & Nass, R. (1988): Drawing ability in four young children with congenital unilateral brain lesions. *Neuropsychologia* **26,** 359–371.

Teuber, H.L. (1975): Recovery of function after brain injury in Man. *Ciba. Found. Symp.* **34,** 159–190.

Thal, D.J., Marchman, V., Stiles, J., *et al.* (1991): Early lexical development in children with focal brain injury. *Brain Lang.* **40,** 491–527.

Tillema, J.M., Byars, A.W., Jacola, L.M., *et al.* (2008): Cortical reorganization of language functioning following perinatal left MCA stroke. *Brain Lang.* **105,** 99–111.

Van Buuren, L.M., van der Aa, N.E., Dekker, H.C., *et al.* (2013): Cognitive outcome in childhood after unilateral perinatal brain injury. *Dev. Med. Child Neurol.* **55,** 934–940.

Vargha-Khadem, F., Isaacs, E., van der Werf, S., Robb, S. & Wilson, J. (1992): Development of intelligence and memory in children with hemiplegic cerebral palsy. The deleterious consequences of early seizures. *Brain* **115,** 315–329.

Vicari, S., Albertoni, A., Chilosi, A.M., Cipriani, P., Cioni, G. & Bates, E. (2000): Plasticity and reorganization during language development in children with early brain injury. *Cortex* **36**(1), 31–46.

Westmacott, R., Askalan, R., MacGregor, D., Anderson, P. & Deveber, G. (2010): Cognitive outcome following unilateral arterial ischaemic stroke in childhood: effects of age at stroke and lesion location. *Dev. Med. Child Neurol.* **52,** 386–393.

(Reid *et al.*, 2014). Cognitive findings in spastic bilateral diplegia are different from those with unilateral involvement, however, a comparison between the neuro-cognitive profiles of these forms has not been proposed.

Most studies of bilateral CP have been conducted in children with diplegia and have underlined a neuro-cognitive picture characterized by a low performance intelligence quotient; normal verbal abilities, impairments in neuro-visual abilities, and high frequency learning difficulties.

Cognitive profile

Abercrombie and colleagues (1964) first described the typical pattern of cognitive impairment in spastic diplegic children in the 1960s. The authors found a greater involvement of visuo-motor and perceptual abilities (performance IQ) in spite of a better verbal quotient using the Wechsler Intelligence Scales (Wechsler, 1949) and they hypothesized that this pattern was related to oculo-motor disorders, such as strabismus and to 'motor handicap'.

In the 1990s, Fedrizzi and colleagues systematically defined the intellectual profile of diplegic children. In a sample of 30 preterm children with spastic diplegia, the pattern of cognitive impairment described using the Wechsler Scales (Wechsler, 1974, 1986) was characterized by a significant difference between the mean verbal IQ, within normal range, and the mean performance IQ, which was lower (Fedrizzi *et al.*, 1996). These data were very similar to those reported in their previous studies (Fedrizzi *et al.*, 1993) and indicated that the neuropsychological profile of preterm children with diplegia is characterized by a specific failure in visuo-perceptual functions. Moreover, only performance IQ was negatively correlated with the typical MRI features of periventricular leukomalacia (PVL), such as the severity of ventricular dilatation, the involvement of white matter, corpus callosum, and optic radiation.

Pagliano and colleagues (2007) investigated cognitive and visuo-perceptual profile in 24 children with spastic diplegia and PVL, using the Griffiths Development Scales (Griffiths, 1984). Developmental Quotient was substantially similar in children born preterm and at term and it was characterized by a discordant neuro-developmental profile, with hearing and speech scores significantly better than performance scores, which were correlated to the severity of PVL.

A debate has concerned the relationship between the typical cognitive pattern with lower levels of performance IQ and visuo-spatial abilities. Many authors have stressed that performance IQ should not be considered a measure of visuo-perceptual abilities, because success in these intellectual tests is also dependent on the integrity of other cognitive integrative functions, as Stiers and colleagues have tried to demonstrate in their studies (Stiers *et al.*, 1999, 2002).

Visual and visuo-cognitive profile

CP children present numerous disorders involving the visual system. The spectrum of visual disorders is extremely broad and includes both peripheral problems (such as strabismus, refraction disorders, and retinopathies) and cerebral visual impairment (CVI), a deficit of visual function caused by damage to, or malfunctioning of, the retrogeniculate visual pathways (optic radiations, occipital cortex, and visual associative areas) in the absence of any major ocular disease (Fazzi *et al.*, 2007, 2012a).

A recent study (Fazzi *et al.*, 2012b) of 129 children with spastic CP documented that children with diplegic CP had, above all, refractive errors, strabismus, abnormal saccadic movements, and reduced visual acuity. Subjects with hemiplegia mainly presented refractive errors, strabismus, and reduced visual field (oculomotor involvement was less frequent), while participants with tetraplegia showed a severe visual impairment characterized by ocular abnormalities, oculomotor dysfunctions, and reduced visual acuity. Cerebral visual impairment appears to be related to the severity of the motor and cognitive impairment as well as the presence of epilepsy (Dufresne et al., 2014).

Since the definition by Good in 2001 (Good, 2001), the clinical spectrum of CVI has been extended to include cognitive visual dysfunctions (CVDs) which are linked to impairment of the higher functions required to analyze and process visual information. These can also constitute the main clinical expressions of CVI in subjects with normal or near-normal visual acuity/visual field and are related to malfunctioning of the occipito-temporal system (the ventral stream, that permits functional and semantic recognition of visual targets) and/or the occipito-parietal system (the dorsal stream, that is specialized in non-conscious visually-guided action planning).

The main clinical features of CVDs in CP arise especially during school age and involve difficulties in writing graphemes, establishing the correct pencil grip, reading with diminishing print size, using scissors, buttoning up buttons, and building with construction toys. Patients also complain about an aching hand while writing, misusing lines and margins, and making inappropriately-sized and spaced letters. The common presence of these dysfunctions partially accounts for the various issues described by school-aged CP children that often involve academic competences.

The visuo-spatial impairment related to dorsal stream damage has been well documented in the literature, and it has long been considered the hallmark of CVDs, nevertheless, some recent studies also report difficulties involving object recognition. Stiers and colleagues (2001) reported that subjects with early cerebral damage can recognize forms, but they fail in the recognition of objects presented in an unusual way. Fazzi and collaborators (2004) observed a deficit in the incomplete figure recognition test in preterm subjects with PVL, which could be interpreted as a difficulty in gestalt perception related to ventral stream processing. In a more recent study (Fazzi et al., 2009), the authors assessed higher visual abilities in a sample of children with PVL and spastic diplegia and observed a widespread impairment of higher visual processing, involving both the ventral and the dorsal visual systems. This pattern supports the idea of integration between the two pathways even if a correlation between the visuo-cognitive profile and structural brain lesions has not yet been identified. Fazzi and colleagues (2009) hypothesized that visuo-cognitive impairments may depend on atypical processing of information in a widespread network of brain areas, which will not necessarily be detected by structural brain imaging, but linked to the well-known problem of brain disconnectivity which is at the basis of preterm encephalopathy (Volpe, 2009).

Language

Speech and language disorders are one of the major associated symptoms in children with CP (Bishop et al., 1987; Love et al., 1980; Luoma et al., 1998). Children with severely limited motor abilities and lower intellectual capacity have lower levels of communication skills (van Schie et al., 2013).

The prevalence of language disorders is still unclear because it depends on the type of CP, on the language skills evaluated, and on the age of the subjects at the moment of evaluation. In children with CP, language difficulties generally appear to decrease in older ages, while social disfunction and communication restrictions appear to increase into adolescence and adulthood. In a recent study, Hustad and collaborators (2013) found that 85 per cent of 2-year-old children with bilateral and unilateral CP had clinical speech and/or language delays relative to age expectations. In a group of adolescents, aged 16-18 years, with bilateral CP, 63 per cent had impaired speech of varying severity. Most of them had been provided with augmentative and alternative communication (AAC), but few used it for communication (Cockerill, 2014).

The most described language impairment concerns speech function, due to a disturbed neuromuscular control of speech mechanism (Pennington & McConachie, 2001a, 2001b; Pirila *et al.*, 2004). Its prevalence remains variable with percentages ranging from 36 to 80 per cent of children with spastic CP (Chen *et al.*, 2010; Odding *et al.*, 2006; Parkes, 2010; Peeters *et al.*, 2008). Even in children who have an IQ above 70, motor speech problems are still present (Pirila *et al.*, 2007). Such problems also impair functional communication skills. Pirila and colleagues (2007) underline that these patients rarely initiate exchange in conversation with adults, take fewer turns in conversation relative to their adult partners and often fail to reply, tend to reply simply using 'yes/no' answers, and rarely ask questions (Basil, 1992; Light *et al.*, 1985b; Pennington, 1999; Pennington & McConachie, 1999).

As far as narrative abilities are concerned, difficulties in relating the sequence of story events and their temporal relationships are also associated with speech problems. The results of a study by Holck and collaborators (2011) indicate a general problem with cohesion at the textual level in a CP group.

Speech and language treatment can be a complex intervention since CP children have complex communication disorders that require different types of treatment. In addition, children who come from different environments are likely to have different social relationships and scholastic experiences, which will influence their language skills and thus their treatment. There is no single universally appropriate form of speech and language therapy. Intervention can focus on speech, expressive or receptive language development, or helping children to develop conversation skills, such as asking questions and repairing conversation in the event of misunderstanding. However, there are no concordant results with regards to effectiveness of these therapeutic approaches.

Pennington and colleagues (2004) analyzed different forms of language training, some of which focused on children (targeted pre-intentional communication skills, the use of individual communicative functions, expressive language, receptive vocabulary, and speech production) while others concentrated on adult conversational partners (teaching them to use communication using an augmentative communication system). However, confirming the effectiveness of language therapies focused either on children or on adults was not possible because of the heterogeneous and poorly described samples included in the analysis, as well as the different aims and methods of therapies.

Suggestions about the utility of further research to describe language profile in CP and to analyze the treatments currently used in speech and language therapy still remain a permanent feature in the conclusions of most of the studies examined.

Learning difficulties in cerebral palsy

Given the high prevalence of learning difficulties in CP children, only few studies have attempted to examine this issue in detail, with sparse results regarding the profile of components involved (Anderson, 1973; Frampton *et al.*, 1998; Schenker *et al.*, 2005).

In a study addressing the interrelationship between the components of health within the inclusive school context, Schenker and colleagues (2005) reported that 46 per cent of CP children (of whom 50 per cent were diplegic) had learning difficulties, the most common additional impairment in the clinical sample described by the authors.

Frampton and colleagues (1998) investigated learning difficulties in children with hemiplegic CP attending special or regular schools and found that 36 per cent had at least one learning difficulty, with major involvement of the arithmetic component (25 per cent of the sample) and less involvement of reading abilities.

Given the lack of insight into the cause, the need to examine the possible origins of learning difficulties has led some authors to investigate to what extent this clinical population is at risk of impairment of academic performances.

Reading disorders

With regards to reading disorders, some authors have investigated the precursors of word decoding in patients with CP (Dahlgren & Sandberg, 2006; Peeters et al., 2009a, 2009b; Pirila et al., 2007). Given the high percentage of dysarthria in this clinical population, they attempted to define the role of articulatory ability in the development of phonological processing. Approximately 20 per cent of CP children are unable to produce intelligible speech (Chan et al., 2005; Pennington et al., 2005). According to Baddeley and Hitch's theory (1974), special attention has been paid to the role of speech production skills in the development of phonological awareness and word decoding. The phonological loop plays an important role in learning phoneme-grapheme conversion rules necessary for word decoding and ultimately text comprehension (Baddeley, 2003).

Several studies have demonstrated that children with CP lag behind in their verbal working memory (WM) skills (Dahlgren & Sandberg, 2006; Peeters et al., 2008), which might have consequences for their reading development. Moreover, Peeters and colleagues (2009) demonstrated that CP children with additional intellectual and speech impairments are at risk of limited verbal working memory spans. However, until now, it is not clear how the additional speech and intellectual impairments play a role in the development of verbal WM in CP children.

While a good deal of recent research has focused on the role of phonological skills in learning written language (Goswami & Bryant, 1990; Muter et al., 1997; Rack et al., 1993), little attention has been given to developmental changes in the way visual information is extracted from print.

Reading comprises several functional components (Marshall & Newcombe, 1973) which range from visual/orthographic processing at early stages to phonological and semantic processing at later stages, and this process takes many years to be acquired (Aghababian & Nazir, 2000). At early visual/orthographic levels of coding, words are thought to pass through a series of hierarchically organised processing steps that start with the elaboration of simple visual features, followed by increasingly larger visual units, from single letters to entire words (Vinckier et al., 2007; Dehaene et al., 2004a). In particular, Dehaene and colleagues (2005) detected a redundant repertoire of reading-related neurons that form a hierarchy of local combination detectors, sensitive to increasingly larger fragments of words.

Reading is thus also a visual task and the way visual information is extracted from print may be shaped by the purpose of the reader to recognize the word. Several studies have suggested that difficulties in the visuo-attentive control system can lead to difficulties, both in the recognition of the feature position and in reading non-words (Cestnick & Coltheart, 1999).

Stein (2001) demonstrated that ocular-motor disorders can impair early reading skills. CP children, in the absence of severe intellectual disability, have disturbed visual skills and visual perception that usually leads to reading difficulties. It is also suggested that microsaccadic skills of CP children is an identifiable adverse factor influencing reading abilities. Moreover, Rosazza and colleagues (Rosazza et al., 2009) found that ventral occipito-temporal and dorsal occipito-parietal pathways cooperate during visual word recognition and assert that processing in these pathways should not be considered as an alternative, but as complementary elements of reading. Andrews and collaborators (2010) found a correlation between preterm birth, damage to white matter and reading skills. All these data suggest the hypothesis of a major susceptibility to reading difficulties in CP children who present a major vulnerability to damage in the areas mentioned, even though no correlational studies are available.

Arithmetic disorders

Compared to their peers with normal development, children with CP are generally delayed in arithmetic performance. During the last 10 years, a few authors have demonstrated interest in the origins of arithmetic impairment, even though no studies have addressed only bilateral spastic forms. Different cognitive factors appear to influence early numeracy abilities; cognitive competences, motor factors, working memory components, and visuo-spatial abilities (Van Rooijen et al., 2014).

With regards to cognitive competences, a positive correlation between non-verbal intelligence and the ability to solve addition and subtraction tasks during primary school was identified (Van Rooijen, et al., 2011). Moreover, non-verbal intelligence appears to be strongly related to early numeracy skills which are predictive of the arithmetic accuracy of children with CP in mainstream and special education programs (2007).

Arithmetic difficulties in CP have been also considered an indirect consequence of neuromotor deficits that characterize such a clinical profile. The studies of Jenks and colleagues (2007, 2009a, 2009b) showed that CP subjects have difficulties in simple arithmetic (multiplying, subtracting, and addition up to 10) and need to use an immature strategy of counting that does not allow them to overcome their evident motor difficulties.

The relationship between working memory and arithmetic performances has largely been studied also in children with normal development. Jenks and collaborators (2007) found a strong relationship between the Baddeley and Hitch visuo-spatial sketchpad (Baddeley & Hitch, 1974), arithmetic accuracy, and simple addition/subtraction reaction times in a sample of children with unilateral and bilateral spastic CP. Rasmussen and Bisanz (2005) have hypothesized that this correlation reflects difficulties to maintain a non-verbal representation of numbers in WM. It can also reflect difficulties to temporarily preserve the position of a number on the mental number line (Barth et al., 2006).

Visuo-spatial problems can also be related to calculation problem solving. Arp and colleagues (2006) hypothesized that difficulties in subityzing (the ability to identify the quantity of a certain amount of items that are presented in too short a time to make counting possible) (Desoete et al., 2009) are related to impaired visuo-spatial analysis of the environment.

Research on adults have furthermore confirmed the presence of contiguity and/or overlap between the areas of calculation and visuo-spatial representation (Dehaene et al., 2004b, Dehaene, 2009). This overlap is particularly significant in CP children with a damaged dorsal pathway. This evidence reinforces the belief in specific calculation disturbances and raises relevant problems from a clinical-diagnostic and rehabilitative point of view.

Conclusion

This review has shown how neuropsychological dysfunctions are an integral part of the clinical picture of CP and how they contribute to characterize the nature of this neurological pathology. The neuro-cognitive disorders that come to light in bilateral spastic CP are strictly correlated, from a functional and neuro-anatomical point of view, with relevant implications in clinical practice. A complete neuropsychological evaluation appears to be essential in subjects with spastic diplegia who usually present a normal total IQ and are adequately scholarized. Given the relevant consequences of rehabilitation programs, this evaluation should accompany traditional motor and cognitive diagnostic procedures, despite the time-consuming limit represented by the long duration of the assessment batteries.

During school age, the neuromotor rehabilitation therapies stop to have a primary role. Identifying new rehabilitation programs tailored to these specific weaknesses and based on the promotion of visuo-cognitive strategies and imitation, becomes more and more urgent, as supported by recent neuroscience research in the last few years.

Conflicts of interest: none.

References

Abercrombie, M.L.J., Gardiner, P.A., Hansen, E., Jonckheere, J., Lindon, R.L., Solomon, G. & Tyson, M.C. (1964): Visual perceptual and visuomotor impairment in physically handicapped children. *Percept. Mot. Skills.* **18,** 561–625.

Aghababian V. & Nazir T.A. (2000): Developing normal reading skills: aspects of the visual processes underlying word recognition. *J. Exp. Child Psychol.* **76,** 123–150.

Anderson, E.M. (1973): *The disabled school child. a study of integration in primary schools.* London, Methuen & Co.

Andrews, J.S., Shachar, M.B., Yeatman, J.D., Flom, L., Luna, B. & Feldman, H.M. (2010): Reading performance correlates with white matter properties in preterm and term children. *Dev. Med. Child Neurol.* **52,** 94–100.

Arp, S., Taranne, P. & Fagard, J. (2006): Global perception of small numerosities (subitizing) in cerebral-palsied children. *J. Clin. Exp. Neuropsychol.* **28,** 405–419.

Baddeley, A. (2003): Working memory and language: an overview. *J. Commun. Disord.* **36**: 189–208.

Baddeley A.D. & Hitch, G.J. (1974): Working memory. In: *The psychology of learning and motivation: advances in research and theory.* eds, G.H. Bower. New York: Academic Press.

Barth, H., La Mont, K., Lipton, J., Dehaene, S., Kanwisher, N. & Spelke, E. (2006): Non-symbolic arithmetic in adults and young children. *Cognition* **98**(3), 199–222.

Basil, C. (1992). Social interaction and learned helplessness in severely disabled children. *Augmentative and Alternative Communication* **8,** 188–199.

Bax, M., Goldstein, M., Rosenbaum, P., Levinton, A., Paneth, N., Dan, B., Jacobsson, B. & Damiano D.(2005): Proposed definition and classification of cerebral palsy. *Dev. Med. Child Neurol.* **47,** 571–576.

Bishop, D.V.M. (1987): The causes of specific developmental language disorder. *J. Child Psychol. Psychiatry* **28,** 1–218.

Cestnick, L. & Coltheart, M. (1999): The relationship between language-processing and visual-processing deficits in developmental dyslexia. *Cognition* **71**(3), 231–255.

Chan, H.S., Lau, P.H., Fong, K.H., Poon, D. & Lam, C.C. (2005): Neuroimpairment, activity limitation, and participation restriction among children with cerebral palsy in Hong Kong. *Hong Kong Med. J.* **11,** 342–350.

Chen, C.L., Lin, K.C., Chen, C.H., Chen, C.C., Liu, W.Y., Chung, C.Y., Chen, C.Y. & Wu, C.Y. (2010): Factors associated with motor speech control in children with spastic cerebral palsy. *Chang Gung Med. J.* **33**(4), 415–423.

Cockerill, H., Elbourne, D., Allen, E., Scrutton, D., Will, E., McNee, A., Fairhurst, C. & Baird, G. (2014): Speech, communication and use of augmentative communication in young people with cerebral palsy: the SH&PE population study. *Child Care Health Dev.* **40**(2), 149–157.

Dahlgren Sandberg, A. (2006): Reading and spelling abilities in children with severe speech impairments and cerebral palsy at 6, 9, and 12 years of age in relation to cognitive development: a longitudinal study. *Dev. Med. Child Neurol.* **48,** 629–634.

Dehaene, S. (2009): Origins of mathematical intuitions: the case of arithmetic. *Ann. N. Y. Acad. Sci.* **1156,** 232–259.

Dehaene, S., Jobert, A., Naccache, L., Ciuciu, P., Poline, J.B., Le Bihan, D. & Cohen, L. (2004a): Letter biding and invariant recognition of masked words: behavioral and neuroimaging evidence. *Psychol. Sci.* **15,** 307–313.

Dehaene, S., Molko, N., Cohen, L. & Wilson, A.J. (2004b): Arithmetic and the brain. *Current Opin. Neurobiol.* **14,** 218–224.

Dehaene, S., Cohen, L., Sigman, M. & Vinckier, F. (2005): The neural code for written words: a proposal. *Trends Cogn. Sci.* **9,** 335–341.

Desoete, A., Ceulemans, A., Roeyers, H. & Huylebroeck, A. (2009). Subitizing or counting as possible screening variables for learning disabilities in mathematics education or learning? *Ed. Res. Rev.* **4,** 55–66.

Dufresne, D., Dagenais, L. & Shevell, M.I. (2014): Spectrum of Visual Disorders in a Population-Based Cerebral Palsy Cohort. *Pediatr. Neurol.* **50**(4), 324–328.

Fazzi, E., Bova, S.M., Uggetti, C., Signorini, S.G., Bianchi, P.E., Maraucci I., Zoppello, M. & Lanzi, G. (2004): Visual-perceptual impairment in children with periventricular leukomalacia. *Brain Dev.* **26**(8), 506–512.

Fazzi, E., Signorini S.G., Bova S.M., La Piana R., Ondei P., Bertone C., Misefari W., Bianchi P.E. (2007): Spectrum of visual disorders in children with cerebral visual impairment. *J Child Neurol.* **22**(3), 294-301.

Fazzi, E., Bova, S., Giovenzana, A., Signorini, S., Uggetti, C. & Bianchi, P.E. (2009): Cognitive visual dysfunction in preterm children with periventricular leukomalacia. *Dev. Med. Child Neurol.* **51,** 974–981.

Fazzi, E., Galli, J. & Micheletti, S. (2012a): Visual impairment: a common sequela of preterm birth. *NeoReviews* **13**(9), e542–550.

Fazzi, E., Signorini, S.G., La Piana, R., Bertone, C., Misefari, W., Galli, J., Balottin, U. & Bianchi, P.E. (2012b): Neuro-ophthalmological disorders in cerebral palsy: ophthalmological, oculomotor, and visual aspects. *Dev. Med. Child Neurol.* **54**(8), 730–736.

Fedrizzi, E., Inverno, M., Botteon, G., Anderloni, A., Filippini, G. & Farinotti, M. (1993): The cognitive development of children born preterm and affected by spastic diplegia. *Brain Dev.* **15**(6), 428–432.

Fedrizzi, E., Inverno, M., Bruzzone, M.G., Botteon, G., Saletti, V. & Farinotti, M. (1996): MRI features of cerebral lesions and cognitive functions in preterm spastic diplegic children. *Pediatr. Neurol.* **15,** 207–212.

Frampton, I., Yude, C. & Goodman, R. (1998): The prevalence and correlates of specific learning difficulties in a representative sample of children with hemiplegia. *Brit. J. Ed. Psychol.* **68,** 39–51.

Good, W.V., Jan, J.E., Burden, S.K., Skoczenski, A. & Candy, R. (2001): Recent advances in cortical visual impairment. *Dev. Med. Child Neurol.* **43**(1), 56–60.

Goswami, U. & Bryant P. (1990): Phonological Skills and Learning to Read (Essays in *Developmental Psychology*). Hove: Psychology Press.

Griffiths, R. (1984): The Abilities of Young Children: A Comprehensive System of Mental Measurement for the First Eight Years of Life. High Wycombe: Test Agency.

Holck, P., Dahlgren Sandberg, A. & Nettelbladt, U. (2011): Narrative ability in children with cerebral palsy. *Res. Dev. Disabil.* **32,** 262–270.

Hustad, K.C., Allison, K., McFadd, E. & Riehle, K. (2013): Speech and language development in 2-year-old children with cerebral palsy. *Dev. Neurorehabil.* **17**(3), 167–175.

Jenks, K.M., De Moor, J., van Lieshout, E.C.D.M., Maathuis, K.G.B., Keus, I. & Gorter, J.W. (2007): The effect of cerebral palsy on arithmetic accuracy is mediated by working memory, intelligence, early numeracy and instruction time. *Dev. Neuropsychol.* **32,** 861–879.

Jenks K.M., deMoor, J. & van Lieshout, E.C.D.M. (2009a): Arithmetic difficulties in children with cerebral palsy are related to executive function and working memory. *J. Child Psychol. Psychiatry.* **50,** 824–833.

Jenks, K.M., van Lieshout, E.C.D.M. & de Moor, J. (2009b): The relationship between medical impairments and arithmetic development in children with cerebral palsy. *J. Child Neurol.* **24,** 528–535.

Light, J., Collier, B. & Parnes, P. (1985b). Communicative interaction between young non-speaking physically disabled children and their primary caregivers. Part II. Communicative function. *Augmentative and Alternative Communication* **1,** 98–107.

Love, R.J., Hagerman, E.L. & Taimi, E.G. (1980): Speech performance, dysphagia and oral reflexes in cerebral palsy. *J. Speech Hear. Disord.* **45,** 59-75.

Luoma, L., Herrgard, E., Martikainen, A. & Ahonen, T. (1998): Speech and language development of children born at 32 weeks' gestation: A 5-year prospective follow-up study. *Dev. Med. Child Neurol.* **40,** 380–387.

Marshall, J.C. & Newcombe, F. (1973): Patterns of paralexia: a psycholinguistic approach. *J. Psycholinguist Res.* **2**(3), 175–199.

Muter, V., Hulme, C., Snowling, M. & Taylor, S. (1997): Segmentation, not rhyming, predicts early progress in learning to read. *J. Exp. Child Psychol.* **65**(3), 370–396.

Odding, E., Roebroeck, M.E. & Stam, H.J. (2006): The epidemiology of cerebral palsy: incidence, impairments and risk factors. *Disabil. Rehabil.* **28**(4), 183–191.

Pagliano, E., Fedrizzi, E., Erbetta, A., Bulgheroni, S., Solari, A., Bono, R., Fazzi, E., Andreucci, E. & Riva, D. (2007): Cognitive profiles and visuoperceptual abilities in preterm and term spastic diplegic children with periventricular leukomalacia. *J. Child Neurol.* **22**(3), 282–288.

Parkes, J., Hill, N., Platt, M.J. & Donnelly, C. (2010): Oromotor dysfunction and communication impairments in children with cerebral palsy: a register study. *Dev. Med. Child Neurol.* **52**, 1113–1119.

Peeters, M., Verhoeven, L., van Balkom, H. & de Moor, J. (2008): Foundations of phonological awareness in pre-school children with cerebral palsy: the impact of intellectual disability. *J. Intellect. Disabil. Res.* **52**(1), 68–78.

Peeters, M., Verhoeven, L. & de Moor, J. (2009a): Predictors of verbal working memory in children with cerebral palsy. *Res. Dev. Disabil.* **30**, 1502–1511.

Peeters, M., Verhoeven, L., de Moor, J., van Balkom, H. (2009b). Importance of speech production for phonological awareness and word decoding: The case of children with cerebral palsy. *Res. Dev. Disabil.* **30**, 712–726.

Pennington, L. (1999): Assessing the communication skills of children with cerebral palsy: does speech intelligibility make a difference? *Child Lang. Teach. Therapy* **15**, 159–169.

Pennington, L. & McConachie, H. (1999): Mother–child interaction revisited: communication with non-speaking physically disabled children. *Int. J. Lang. Commun. Disord.* **34**, 391–416.

Pennington, L. & McConachie, H. (2001a). Interaction between children with cerebral palsy and their mothers: the effects of speech intelligibility. *Int. J. Lang. Commun. Disord.* **36**, 371–393.

Pennington, L. & McConachie, H. (2001b). Predicting patterns of interaction between children with cerebral palsy and their mothers. *Dev. Med. Child Neurol.* **43**, 83–90.

Pennington, L., Goldbart, J. & Marshall, J. (2004) Speech and language therapy to improve the communication skills of children with cerebral palsy. *Cochrane Database of Systematic Reviews* **3**, CD003466.

Pennington, L., Goldbart, J. & Marshall J. (2005): Direct speech and language therapy for children with cerebral palsy: findings from a systematic review. *Dev. Med. Child Neurol.* **47**, 57–63.

Pirila, S., van der Meere, J., Korhonen, P., Ruusu-Niemi, P., Kyntaja, M., Nieminen, P. & Korpela, R. (2004): A retrospective neurocognitive study in children with spastic diplegia. *Dev. Neuropsychol.* **26**(3), 679–90.

Pirila, S., van der Meere, J., Pentikainen, T., Ruusu-Niemi, P., Korpela, R., Kilpinen, J. & Nieminen, P. (2007): Language and motor speech skills in children with cerebral palsy. *J. Commun. Disord.* **40**, 116–128.

Rack, J.P., Hulme, C. & Snowling, M.J. (1993): Learning to read: a theoretical synthesis. *Adv. Child Dev. Behav.* **24**, 99–132.

Rasmussen, C. & Bisanz, J. (2005): Representation and working memory in early arithmetic. *J. Exp. Child Psychol.* **91**(2), 137–157.

Reid, S.M., Dagia, C.D., Ditchfield, M.R., Carlin, J.B. & Reddihough, D.S. (2014): Population-based studies of brain imaging patterns in cerebral palsy. *Dev. Med. Child Neurol.* **56**, 222–232.

Rosazza, C., Cai, Q., Minati, L., Paulignan, Y. & Nazir, T. (2009): Early development of dorsal and ventral pathways in visual word recognition: an ERP study. *Brain Res.* **1272**, 32–44.

Schenker, R., Coster, W.J. & Parush, S. (2005): Neuroimpairments, activity performance, and participation in children with cerebral palsy mainstreamed in elementary schools. *Dev. Med. Child Neurol.* **47**, 808–814.

Stein, J. (2001): The magnocellular theory of development dyslexia. *Dyslexia* **7**, 12–36.

Stiers, P., De Cock, P. & Vandenbussche, E. (1999). Separating visual perception and non-verbal intelligence in children with early brain injury. *Brain Dev.* **21**, 397–406.

Stiers, P., van den Hout, B.M., Haers, M., Vanderkelen, R., de Vries, L.S., van Nieuwenhuizen, O. & Vandenbussche, E. (2001): The variety of visual perceptual impairments in pre-school children with perinatal brain damage. *Brain Dev.* **23**(5), 333–348.

Stiers, P., Vanderkelen, R., Vanneste, G., Coene, S., De Rammelaere, M. & Vandenbussche, E. (2002): Visual-perceptual impairment in a random sample of children with cerebral palsy. *Dev. Med. Child Neurol.* **44**: 370–382.

Van Rooijen, M., Verhoeven, L. & Steenbergen, B. (2011): Early numeracy in cerebral palsy: review and future research. *Dev. Med. Child Neurol.* **53**, 202–209.

Van Rooijen, M., Verhoeven, L., Smits, D.W., Dallmeijer, A.J., Becher, J.G. & Steenbergen, B. (2014): Cognitive precursors of arithmetic development in primary school children with cerebral palsy. *Res. Dev. Disabil.* **35**, 826–832.

Van Schie, P.E., Siebes, R.C., Dallmeijer, A.J., Schuengel, C., Smits, D.W., Gorter, J.W. & Becher, J.G. (2013): Development of social functioning and communication in school-aged (5-9 years) children with cerebral palsy. *Res. Dev. Disabil.* **34**(12), 4485–4494.

Vinckier, F., Dehaene, S., Jobert, A., Dubus, J.P., Sigman, M. & Cohen, L. (2007): Hierarchical coding of letter strings in the ventral stream: dissecting the inner organization of the visual word-form system. *Neuron* **55**(1), 143–156.

Volpe, J.J. (2009): Brain injury in premature infants: a complex amalgam of destructive and developmental disturbances. *Lancet Neurol.* **8,** 110–124.

Wechsler, D. (1949): *Wechsler Intelligence Scale for Children*. New York: Psychological Corp.

Wechsler, D. (1974): *Manuale della Scala Wechsler a Livello Prescolare e di Scuola Elementare (WPPSI)*. Firenze: O.S. Organizzazioni Speciali.

Wechsler, D. (1986): *Manuale della Scala di Intelligenza Wechsler per Bambini-Riveduta (WISC-R)*. Firenze: O.S. Organizzazioni Speciali.

Progressive neurological diseases

Chorea

Chorea is an ongoing, random-appearing sequence of one or more involuntary movements (Sanger et al., 2010).

Sydenham chorea

Sydenham chorea is estimated to occur in 10 to 30 per cent of children with rheumatic fever. Retrospective studies based on medical charts indicate that 46 per cent of children exhibit behavioural changes; parents describe emotional liability, irritability, and age-regressed behaviour (Swedo et al., 1993). Obsessive compulsive (OC) symptoms have been extensively described with different time courses. Two prospective studies using formal psychiatric evaluation (Diagnostic and Statistical Manual of Mental Disorders, 3rd Edition, Revised and Leyton Obsessional Inventory Child Version) demonstrated an association with OC symptoms (70-80 per cent); some patients met the OCD (Obsessive compulsive disorder) criteria (17-27 per cent) (Maia et al., 2005; De Alvarenga et al., 2009; Asbahr et al., 1998). OC symptoms which were present only in children with Sydenham chorea, and not in children with rheumatic fever, peaked during the acute phase after the first two months and disappeared at six months. Another systematic study, using DSM-IV criteria, reported that OCD was not significant in the acute phase of the disease, but was found in 50 per cent of children with persistent Sydenham chorea (Maia et al., 2005). Common compulsions were checking, cleaning, and repeating actions; the two most reported symptoms were aggressive behaviour and fear of contamination (Asbahr et al., 2005). In addition, a retrospective study described depression during and after Sydenham symptoms, and anxiety before, during, and after clinical symptoms (Ridel et al., 2010). A prospective controlled study found that individuals with Sydenham chorea have a higher risk of developing schizophrenia (Wilcox & Nasrallah, 1988). Cognitive deficits are also present in this movement disorder: ADHD symptoms, lower scores on the Weschler Intelligence Scale for Children-Revised, and impaired verbal fluency, attributed to frontal lobe dysfunction (Ridel et al., 2010; Swedo et al., 1993; Cunningham et al., 2006).

Benign hereditary chorea

Benign hereditary chorea is a familial dominant disorder related to a mutation in the thyroid transcription factor 1 (*TIFF1*) gene with thyroid and lung involvement. Some patients affected have a low IQ. There are no reports of cognitive decline (Bird et al., 1976; Kleiner-Firsman & Lang, 2007).

Myoclonus

Myoclonus is a sequence of repeated, often non-rhythmic, brief shock-like jerks due to sudden involuntary contraction or relaxation of one or more muscles (Sanger et al., 2010).

Opsoclonus-myoclonus syndrome

Opsoclonus-myoclonus syndrome is a paraneoplastic disorder presenting in infancy with paroxysmal erratic eye movement (opsoclonus), myoclonus, and ataxia. Most studies reported cognitive impairment presenting as developmental delay. The course of the disease frequently leads to a low intellectual capacity (IQ levels between 50 and 70) in the majority of patients, speech impairments (verbal fluency and articulation are impaired whereas verbal comprehension and language pragmatics are preserved), and behavioural problems (persistent irritability, dysphoric mood and poor affective regulation, and aggressive and/or self-injuring behaviours) (Hammer et al., 1995; Koh et al., 1994). Over half of all children require special education. Memory and executive functions are relatively preserved (Papero et al., 1995).

Tourette syndrome

Tics are repeated, intermittent movements which are briefly suppressible and usually associated with a premonitory urge (Sanger et al., 2010).

In Tourette syndrome, vocal and motor tics are present over a year; emotional comorbidities have been studied and described in several reports and are often more disruptive than the tics themselves. ADHD (70 per cent with impaired inhibition and executive function), OCD (26 per cent), separation anxiety (14 per cent), bipolar disorder (11 per cent), depression (2-9 per cent), schizophrenia (3 per cent), and pervasive developmental disorder (5 per cent) have been reported (Burd et al., 2009; Robertson, 2006). In addition, bizarre behaviours, personality disorders, criminal activity, and self-injuring behaviour have been reported in several studies (Ghanizadeb & Mosallaei, 2009). Somato-sensory, compulsive touching and counting and reduced anxiety have been reported more frequently in children with Tourette syndrome and OCD than those with OCD pure. Children with Tourette syndrome usually have a normal IQ, but may present learning disabilities possibly due to an earlier onset and a familial history of tics (Burd et al., 2005).

Children with Tourette syndrome and ADHD have a cognitive profile similar to children with ADHD alone (impaired inhibition and executive function, abnormal visuo-spatial construction, and learning disabilities); children with Tourette syndrome without ADHD exhibit better motor coordination and a higher IQ compared to children with ADHD alone (Denckla, 2006).

Stereotypies

Stereotypies are repeated, repetitive, involuntary movements that may also be rhythmic and continual (Jankovic, 1994); they usually begin within the first 3 years of life, change little over time, and can be voluntarily suppressed. Each individual has his/her own pattern that can evolve over time. In infants and young children, movement ranges from simple thumb/hand sucking and body rocking to more complex motor activities such as head nodding, arm flapping, finger wiggling, and body rocking. Movements appear multiple times a day and are associated with periods of engrossment, excitement, stress, fatigue, or boredom. Motor stereotypies are suppressed by a sensory stimulus or distraction.

Stereotypy movements may be classified into two groups: primary (physiological) and secondary (phatological), depending on the presence of additional signs or symptoms. Primary stereotypies have been reported in several studies of children with normal development (MacDonald et al., 2007; Harris et al., 2008). This category implies that there is not a specific cause and that they occur in a normal individual. Mild early delays in either language or motor development have, however, been noted in some studies (Mahone et al., 2004; Harris et al., 2008). The prevalence of stereotypic movements in typically developing children is unknown; it has been estimated at about 20 per cent (Sallusto & Atwell, 1978). The outcome has been controversial; declining in some studies after the age of four, persisting in others, and present in adults when bored or stressed (MacDonald et al., 2007; Harris et al., 2008; Schalaggar &

Mink, 2003). Secondary stereotypies imply the presence of behavioural or neurological signs and symptoms, associated with autistic spectrum, intellectual disability, sensory deprivation, neurodegenerative disorders, infection, tumour, or psychiatric condition (schizophrenia, OCD). Based on the evaluation of a standardized play session, children with low-functioning autism had a greater prevalence, number, and variety of stereotypies compared to those with high-functioning autism, developmental language disorder, and non-autistic low functioning (Goldman *et al.*, 2009).

Dystonia

Dystonia is an involuntary sustained or intermittent muscle contraction causing twisting and repetitive movements and abnormal postures (Sanger *et al.*, 2010).

Based on aetiology, dystonia can be primary or secondary. Dystonia is the only symptom in primary or idiopathic dystonia; different genes have been identified in primary dystonia, but in several patients, no genetic abnormalities were detected. Secondary dystonia is the result of neurodegenerative diseases, metabolic disorders, or the result a long series of acquired causes. In several studies focusing on the association between dystonia and psychiatric and cognitive disorders, described in adults patients with idiopathic focal dystonia and evaluated by a structured clinical interview (DSM-IV), a fivefold increased risk of psychiatric disorder, frequently presenting before motor manifestations, was reported (Nègre Pagès *et al.*, 2010). Several authors used a detailed assessment of a range of tests evaluating cognitive function (executive function and working memory, including phonemic and semantic word fluency, intellectual ability, language, spatial function, and attention) and did not show any significant deficits, except semantic word fluency (Jahanshahi *et al.*, 2003; Scott *et al.*, 2003). Another study revealed specific deficits based on tests of visual-spatial function relating to egocentric space, semantic verbal fluency, susceptibility to retroactive interference, and deficits in executive function (more perseverative errors relative to controls) (Balas *et al.*, 2006).

Cognition has been also investigated in patients with secondary dystonia suggesting frequent cognitive impairment and dementia. Some studies reported a correlation between adaptive behaviour and the severity of cognitive impairment and motor disabilities (Freeman *et al.*, 2007). Early onset of disease correlated with low intellectual functioning.

Regarding psychiatric symptoms, in dystonia, numerous reports indicate that patients with primary dystonia may have higher rates of depression and anxiety than expected; dysfunctional mood is one of the most important predictors of a patient's quality of life. The prevalence of depression and anxiety varies over the course of a lifetime and in most studies falls in the range of 25 per cent-50 per cent (Jahanshahi & Marsden, 1988, 1990). Patients with mutation in *DYT 1* (with or without symptoms) have a significantly higher rate and earlier onset of major depressive disorders than controls without *DYT 1* mutation (Heiman *et al.*, 2004). Patients suffering from DYT 5 dystonia have a higher rate of depression than the general population (Van Hove *et al.*, 2006). A small group of studies have looked specifically for OC symptoms in dystonia; alcohol abuse and dependence has been reported in myoclonus dystonia linked to *DYT 11* mutation, as well as in primary dystonia (Saunders-Pullman *et al.*, 2002; Hess *et al.*, 2007).

It is not clear whether neuropsychiatric disorders are the result of, or occur independent of, motor manifestations. The underlying pathophysiology of dystonia may predispose patients to mood disorders; striatal pathways involved in mood and behaviour have been shown to be abnormal in functional imaging studies.

Conclusion

Based on the literature, screening for cognitive and psychiatric disorders is important in the evaluation of children suffering from movement disorders; the knowledge of non-motor phenotypes may assist the clinician in management and treatment, and furthermore determine which symptoms are suggestive of a specific movement disorder and which indicate medication effects.

The evaluation should be assessed using a detailed and comprehensive neuropsychological and psychiatric examination, selecting tests that can be performed in adults and children which are less sensitive to test-retest effects and require minimal writing or hand, suitable for patients with severe motor disability.

Since 2011, at the Carlo Besta Neurological Institute of Milan, all child patients with movement disorders complete tests for intellectual capacity and other cognitive functions (language, memory, executive function, attention). General cognitive abilities are assessed using the full intellectual quotient as well as the verbal comprehension index, perceptual reasoning index, working memory index, and processing speed index, and are analyzed by means of the Wechsler Intelligence Scale for children-4th edition (see *Table 1*). In addition, information about behavioural or emotional problems are measured by the Child Behaviour Checklist [CBCL], a parent report measure that yields area scores that are combined to form a total Problems T-score, while the quality of life is investigated using other questionnaires (Child Health Questionnaire; Health Questionnaire SF 36).

Table 1. Neuropsychological Assessment

Intellectual ability	Raven CPM/SPM WPPSI-III/Wisc-IV; WAIS-R Leiter-R
Executive function	Tower of London Verbal fluency Stroop Test Wisconsin's Card
Psychopathology	CBCL 6-18 YSR 11-18/SAFA Beck Depression Inventory-II /Yale-BOCS
Quality of life	Child Health Questionnaire Health Questionnaire SF 36
Language	Peabody Trog-II Verbal Framework NEPSY-II No word list recall
Attention	Barrage (TCM) Continuous Performance Test (BIA) MF
Memory	Digit span Test of Corsi Promea

Conflicts of interest: none.

References

Asbahr, F.R., Garvey, M.A., Snider, L.A., Zanetta, D.M., Elkis, H. & Swedo, S.E. (2005): Obsessive compulsive symptoms among individuals with Sydenham chorea. *Biol. Psychiatry* **57**, 1073–1076.

Asbahr, F.R., Negrao, A.B., Gentil, V., et al. (1998): Obsessive compulsive and related symptoms in children and adolescence with rheumatic fever with and without chorea: a prospective 6-month study. *Am. J. Psychiatry* **155**, 1122–1124.

Balas, M., Perez, C., Badarny, S., Scott, R.B. & Giladi, N. (2006): Neuropsychological profile of DYT 1 dystonia. *Mov. Disord.* **21**, 2073–2077.

Boyle, P.A., Wilson, P.S., Aggarwal, N.T., et al. (2005): Parkinsonian signs in subjects with mild cognitive impairment. *Neurology* **65**, 1901–1906.

Burd, L., Freeman, R.D., Klug, M.G. & Kerbeshian, J. (2005): Tourette syndrome and learning disabilities. *BMC Pediatrics* **5**, 34.

Burd, L., Kerbeshian, J., Klug, M.G. & Freeman, R.D. (2009): Tourette syndrome and comorbid pervasive developmental disorders. *J. Child Neurol.* **24**, 170–175.

Cunningham, M.C., Maia, D.P., Teixeira, A.L. Jr. & Cardoso, F. (2006): Sydenham chorea is associated with decreased verbal fluency. *Parkinsonism Relat. Disord.* **12**, 165–167.

De Alvarenga, P.G., Floresi, A.C., Torres, A.R., et al. (2009): Higher prevalence of obsessive compulsive spectrum disorders in rheumatic fever. *Gen. Hosp. Psychiatry* **31**, 178–180.

Denckla, M.B. (2006): Attention deficit hyperactivity disorder: the childhood co-morbidity that most influences the disability burden in Tourette syndrome. *Adv. Neurol.* **99**, 17–21.

Freeman, K., Gregory, A., Turner, A., Blasco, P., Hogarth, P., Hayflick, S. (2007): Intellectual and adaptive behaviour functioning in panthothenate kinase associated neurodegeneration. *J Intellect Disabil Res.* **51**, 417-426.

Ghanizadeb, A. & Mosallaei, S. (2009): Psychiatric disorders and behavioural problems in children and adolescents with Tourette syndrome. *Brain Dev.* **31**, 15–19.

Goldman, S., Wang, C., Salgado, M.W., Greene, P.E., Kim, M. & Rapin, I. (2009): Motor stereotypies in children with autism and other developmental disorders. *Dev. Med. Child Neurol.* **51**, 30–38.

Hammer, M.S., Larsen, M.B. & Stack, C.V. (1995): Outcome of children with opsoclonus myoclonus regardless of aetiology. *Ped. Neurology* **13**, 21–24.

Harris, K.M., Mahon, E.M. & Singer, H.S. (2008): Non-autistic motor stereotypies: clinical features and longitudinal follow-up. *Ped. Neurology* **38**, 267–272.

Heiman, G.A., Ottman, R., Saunders-Pullman, R.J., Ozelius, L.J., Risch, N.J. & Bressman, S.B. (2004): Increased risk for recurrent major depression in DYT 1 dystonia mutation carriers. *Neurology* **63**, 631–637.

Hess, C.W., Raymond, D., Auuiar Pde, C., et al. (2007): Myoclonus dystonia obsessive compulsive disorder, and alcohol dependence in SGCE mutation carriers. *Neurology* **68**, 522–524.

Jahanshahi, M. & Marsden, C.D. (1988): Personality in torticollis: a controlled study. *Psychol. Med.* **18**, 375–387.

Jahanshahi, M. & Marsden, C.D. (1990): A longitudinal follow-up study of depression, disability and body concept in torcicollis. *Behav. Neurol.* **3**, 233–246.

Jahanshahi, M., Rowe, J. & Fuller, R. (2003): Cognitive executive function in dystonia. *Mov. Disord.* **18**, 1470–1481.

Jankovic J.(1994): stereotypies. In *Movement Disorder 3*, C.D. Marsden, S. Fahn (eds). Oxford: Butterworh-Heinemman, pp. 501–507.

Koh, P.S., Raffensperger, J.G., Berry, S., et al. (1994): Long-term outcome in children with opsoclonus myoclonus and ataxia and coincident neuroblastoma. *J. Pediatr.* **125**, 712–716.

Kuyper, D.J., Parra, V., Aerts, S., Okun, M.S. & Kluger, B.M. (2011): Non-motor manifestation of dystonia: a systematic review. *Mov. Disord.* **26**, 1206–1217.

MacDonald, R., Green, G., Mansfield, R., et al. (2007): Stereotypy in young children with autism and typically developing children. *Res. Dev. Disabil.* **28**, 266–277.

Mahome, E.M., Bridges, D., Prahme, C. & Singer, H.S. (2004): Repetitive arm and hand movement in children. *J. Pediatr.* **145**, 391–395.

Maia, D.P., Teixeira, A.L. Jr, Quintão Cunningham, M.C. & Cardoso, F. (2005): Obssessive compulsive behaviour, hyperactivity, and attention deficit disorders in Sydenham Chorea. *Neurology* **64**, 1799–1801.

Nègre Pagès, L., Grandjen, H., Lapeyre-Mestre, M., et al.; DoPaMiP Study Group. (2010): Anxious and depressive symptoms in Parkinson's disease: the French cross-sectional DoPaMiP study. *Mov. Disord.* **25**, 157–166.

Papero, P.H., Pranzatelli, M.R., Margolis, L.J., Tate, E., Wilson, L.A. & Glass, P. (1995): Neurobehavioral and psychological functioning of children with opsoclonus myoclonus syndrome. *Dev. Med. Child Neurol.* **37,** 915–932.

Ridel, K.R., Lipps, T.D. & Gilbert, D.L. (2010): The prevalence of neuropsychiatric disorders in Sydenham chorea. *Ped. Neurology* **42,** 243–248.

Robertson, M.M. (2006): Mood disorders and Gilles de la Tourette's syndrome: an update on prevalence, aetiology, comorbidity clinical associations and implications. *J. Psychosom. Res.* **61,** 349–358.

Sallusto, F., Atwell, C.W.(1978): Body rocking, head banging and head rolling in normal children. *J Pediatric* **93,** 704-708.

Sanger, T.D., Chen, D., Fehlings, D.L., et al. (2010): Definition and classification of hyperkinetic movement disorders in childhood. *Mov. Disord.* **25,** 1538–1549.

Saunders-Pullman, R., Shriberg, J., Heiman, G., et al. (2002): Myoclonus dystonia: possible association with obsessive compulsive disorder and alcohol dependence. *Neurology* **58,** 242–245.

Schalaggar, B.L. & Mink, J.W. (2003): Movement disorder in children. *Pediatric Rev.* **24,** 39-51.

Scott, R., Gregory, R., Wilson, J., et al. (2003): Executive cognitive deficits in primary dystonia. *Mov. Disord.* **18,** 539–550.

Swedo, S.F., Leonard, H.L., Schapiro, M.B., et al. (1993): Sydenham chorea: physical and psychological symptoms of St Vitus dance. *Pediatrics* **91,** 706–713.

Van Hove, J.L.K., Steyaert, J., Matthijs, G., et al. (2006): Expanded motor and psychiatric phenotype in autosomal dominant Segawa Syndrome due to GTP cyclohydrolase deficiency. *J. Neurol. Neurosurg. Psychiatry* **77,** 18–23.

Wilcox, J.A. & Nasrallah, H. (1988): Sydenham chorea and psychopathology. *Neuropsychobiology* **19,** 6–8.

Test References

Achenbach, T.M. (2001): Child Behavior Checklist for Ages 6-18.

Apolone, G. & Mosconi, P. (1998): The Italian SF 36 Health Survey: Translation, Validation and Norming. *J. Clin. Epidemiol.* **51,** 1025–1036.

Beck, A.T., Steer, R.A. & Brown, G.K. (2006): *BDI-II: Beck Depression Inventory-II*. Ed. O.S. Giunti.

Belacchi, C., Scalisi, T., Cannoni, E. & Cornoldi, C. (2008): *Coloured Progressive Matrices*. Ed. O.S. Giunti.

Bertelli, B. & Bilancia, G. (2006): *VAUMeLF: Batterie per la valutazione dell'attenzione uditiva e della memoria di lavoro fonologica nell'età evolutiva*. Ed. O.S. Giunti.

Bird, R.D., Carlson, C.B. & Hall, J.G. (1976): Familial essential ('benign') chorea. *J. Med. Genet.* **13,** 357–362.

Bishop, D.V.M. (2009): Trog-2: *Test of Reception of Grammar-Version 2*. Ed. O.S. Giunti.

Bisiacchi, P., Cendron, M., Gugliotta, M., Tressoldi, P.E. & Vio, C. (2005): *Batteria di valutazione neuropsicologica per l'età evolutiva*. Ed. Erickson.

Child Health Questionnaire (CHQ PF 50). (2006): Healthact chq. Italian Version.

Cianchetti, C. & Sannio Fancello, G. (2001): *SAFA: Scale psichiatriche di auto somministrazione per fanciulli e adolescenti*. Ed. O.S. Giunti.

Fancello, G., Vio, C. & Cianchetti, C. (2008): *Torre di Londra*. Ed. Erickson.

Goodman, initial. (1989): Scala di Valutazione Ossessivo Compulsiva Yale-Brown Obsessive Compulsive Scale and Symptom Checklist (Y-BOCS).

Heaton, R.K., Chelune, G.J., Talley, J.L., Kay, G.G. & Curtiss, G. (2003): *MCST: Modified Card sorting test*. Ed. O.S. Giunti.

Heaton, R.K., Chelune, G.J., Talley, J.L., Kay, G.G. & Curtiss, G. (2000): *WCST: Wisconsin Card sorting test*. Ed. O.S. Giunti.

Kleiner-Fisman, G. & Lang, A.E. (2007): Benign hereditary chorea revisited: a journey to understanding. *Mov. Disord.* **22,** 2297–2305.

Korkman, M., Kirk, U. & Kemp, S. (2011): *Nepsy-II*. Ed. O.S. Giunti.

Marzocchi, G.M., Re, A.M. & Cornoldi, C. (2010): *Batteria Italiana per L'ADHD*. Ed. Erickson.

Raven, C.J. (2008): *COM: Coloured Progressive Matrices*. Ed. O.S. Giunti.

Raven, C.J. (2008): *Standard Progressive Matrices*. Ed. O.S. Giunti.

Roid, G.H. & Miller, L.J. (2002): *Leiter Intenational Perfomance Scale-Revised*. Ed. O.S. Giunti. Italian edition.

Wechsler, D. (2012): (Adattamento italiano a cura di Orsini, A. & Pezzuti, L., 2012): *Wechsler Intelligence Scale for Children, 4th Edition*. Ed. O.S. Giunti.

Stella, G., Pizzoli, C. & Tressoldi, P. (2000): *Peabody (PPVT)*. Omega Edizioni.
Wechsler, D. (2008): *Wechsler Preschool and Primary Scale of Intelligence, 3rd Edition*. Ed. O.S. Giunti.
Wechsler, D. (1997): *Wechsler Adult Intelligence Scale Revised*. Ed. O.S. Giunti.
Vicari, S. (2007): *PROMEA: prove di memoria e apprendimento per l'età evolutiva*. Ed. O.S. Giunti.

Chapter 17

Lysosomal storage disorders

Rita Barone* and Rossella Parini°

*Unit of Child Neurology and Psychiatry, Policlinico, University of Catania,
via S. Sofia 78, 95123 Catania, Italy;
°Unit of Rare Metabolic Diseases, Paediatric Clinic, San Gerardo Hospital, via Pergolesi 33, 20052 Monza, Italy
rbarone@unict.it, rossella.parini@unimib.it

Summary

The lysosomal storage disorders (LSD) are genetic diseases caused by deficiency of lysosomal enzymes or other lysosomal proteins that result in chronic and progressive storage of undegraded substrates that are frequently present in the central nervous system. Neurocognition in LSD may be impaired with distinct regression or progressive slowing-down of development. The neurological phenotypes of LSD comprise some specific neuropsychological profiles, including verbal and non-verbal learning disorders underlying dysfunction of cerebral networks. Specific behavioural patterns and secondary psychiatric disorders may also occur. The knowledge of certain neuropsychological profiles and behavioural patterns in LSD may be critical for recognition, early diagnosis, and intervention programming and monitoring. Developmental analysis in patients with LSD is hampered by concurrence of physical disability, sensory disturbances, and behavioural abnormalities. The assessment is currently based on evaluation of age-equivalent scores in order to clinically understand developmental progress, stagnation, and loss of abilities in each individual domain. The use of age-equivalent Vineland Adaptive Behaviour Scales is encouraged because of possible discrepancies between cognition and adaptive functioning in patients with impaired motor functions. Neurocognitive assessment of patients with LSD has become increasingly important to define the timing of possible interventions and clinical endpoints. This is crucial in view of emerging treatments of neurogenetic disorders, especially neuronopathic LSD.

Neuronopathic lysosomal storage diseases in childhood

Definition and principles of treatment

The lysosomal storage diseases (LSD) include around 50 diseases described to date and although each of them is rare, their overall prevalence is estimated to be 1 in 7,000 live births (Klein & Futerman, 2013). LSD are caused by mutations in genes encoding catalytic enzymes or enzyme activators, but also in genes that encode lysosomal membrane proteins or proteins involved in enzyme trafficking. Such defects result in chronic and progressive storage of undegraded substrates. The pathophysiology of LSD is unclear but involves an impairment of autophagy, alteration of intracellular calcium homeostasis, activation of signal transduction by non-physiological substances, inflammation, as well as other mechanisms (Bellettato & Scarpa, 2010;

Settembre *et al.*, 2013). Laboratory diagnosis relies on measurements of lysosomal enzyme activities in serum and/or cells, and genotype analyses. LSD present with progressive phenotypes that affect multiple organs and systems, including neurodegeneration. Neurological phenotypes of the primary neuronal forms of LSD are age-related and include an acute infantile deterioration syndrome and late-onset forms. The former is typical of the infantile forms of sphingolipidosis (*i.e.* Gaucher disease type 2, GM1 and GM2 gangliosidosis, Sandhoff disease, and Niemann-Pick disease type A). The acute infantile neuronopathic LSD are characterized by acute psychomotor regression in the first six months of life with axial hypotonia, limb spasticity, increased head circumference, irritability, macular cherry-red spot and blindness, epilepsy, decerebration, and vegetative state. In the late-onset forms, storage phenomena affect several tracts and distinct neurological phenotypes may be observed, including eye movement disorders, pyramidal tract signs, cerebellar dysfunction, epilepsy or myoclonus, and behavioural and psychiatric disturbances (Prada & Grabowski, 2013).

Neuronopathic LSD are a cause of intellectual disability often associated with behavioural problems such as aggressivity, hyperactivity, and self-injuring behaviour. Among genetic diseases that cause intellectual disabilities (ID), inborn errors of metabolism deserve mention because many of them have become amenable to therapy. To overcome the primary deficiency in LSD is theoretically agreeable by correction of the genetic defect, enzyme deficiency, and substrate accumulation (Ortolano *et al.*, 2014). Definition of outcomes of therapy for neuropathic LSD is a major issue because the ideal effect of therapy would be an improvement in IQ and related developmental scores as well as additional co-morbid features such as epilepsy, neurological, behavioural, and psychiatric problems. However, at the time of diagnosis, it is possible that neuronal damage has already occurred, thus the response to treatment is valuable in terms of stabilization or slowing down of progression (Augustine & Mink, 2013). Future perspectives of the treatment of neuronopathic LSD are briefly reported.

Enzyme replacement therapy

A great concern of major clinical relevance is the inability of therapeutic enzymes to cross the blood-brain barrier that makes enzyme replacement therapy (ERT) not recommended for patients with CNS involvement. Currently, enzyme-targetted correction of neuronopathic LSD aims to improve enzyme biodistribution and pharmacokinetic properties, including optimization of enzyme phosphorylation and glycosylation and use of higher dosages or clearance reduction to improve transcytosis through the blood-brain barrier. Enzyme replacement via direct injection into the CNS has been attempted in models of Krabbe disease and mucopolysaccharidosis (MPS) I and IIIA by intrathechal (IT) drug administration or direct intracerebroventricular (ICV) injection (Crawley *et al.*, 2011; Vite *et al.*, 2013).

Widespread distribution and cellular localization of therapeutic enzymes was obtained in the brain after both IT-lumbar and ICV delivery in non-human primates (Calias *et al.*, 2012). Corpus callosum atrophy and white matter changes have been associated with attentive defects and cognitive impairment in human MPS-I (King *et al.*, 2014). IT-ERT prevents corpus callosum atrophy in the canine MPS-I model when early treated (Vite *et al.*, 2013). Corpus callosum volumetric measurements might represent quantitative neuroimaging markers for MPS-related brain disease and its response to therapy.

Clinical trials (phase I/II) have been performed for long-term intrathecal enzyme replacement therapy for patients with MPS type I, II, and IIIA. The trials aim to prevent neurodevelopmental and cognitive impairment associated with MPS. Primary outcome measures are stabilization of cognitive status or slowing the rate of decline of cognitive status, as measured by IQ. Intrathecal enzyme replacement is a promising treatment for the CNS in MPS, but the biochemical data and clinical outcomes are not yet available (Chen *et al.*, 2014).

Haematopoietic stem cell transplantation

Principles of treatment of neuropathic LSD with haematopoietic stem cell transplantation (HSCT) include the possibility that HSCT repopulates the recipient myeloid compartment, including microglia, with cells expressing the defective functional hydrolase. Rate and extent of brain infiltration by transplanted cells relies on several factors, such as the use of a preparatory regimen, presence of a disease state in the brain, and the turnover of transplanted cells with resident microglia.

HSCT has been applied for treatment of some LSD with neurological involvement. For aspartylglucosaminuria, Gaucher disease type III (GD-III), metachromatic leukodystrophy (MLD), and MPS III, HSCT was chosen on an individual basis in the past, but for some diseases it is now considered contraindicated depending also on the age of the patient and clinical picture: globoid cell leukodystrophy with symptomatic early onset, GM1 and GM2 gangliosidosis, early-onset metachromatic leukodystrophy or mucopolysaccharidosis type II already symptomatic with mental delay, MPS III and IV, and Niemann-Pick disease type A, B and C.

It is suggested that in MLD, HSCT might prevent disease progression if performed at a sufficiently early time before loss of walking, which typically initiates rapid deterioration. In infantile Krabbe leukodystrophy, umbilical cord transplantation was effective in asymptomatic patients but had no effects on patients with neurological signs over a 3-year period (van Karnebeek & Stockler, 2012). Conversely, HSCT represents the standard of care in MPS I-Hurler (MPS IH) based on prolongation of survival with therapy, preservation of neurocognition, and amelioration of somatic features. In particular, developmental outcomes are better when the transplant is performed before 24 months of age (de Ru *et al.*, 2011). In MPS I, HSCT is recommended for patients under 2 years of age with normal cognition (DQ < 70). Since 1981, more than 500 MPS I patients have been treated with HSCT. However, owing to the significant morbidity and mortality rate associated with HSCT, ERT remains the primary treatment option for MPS I patients with mild phenotypes or when HSCT cannot be performed.

A recent analyses of HSCT effectiveness in 15 alpha-mannosidosis patients showed that despite the fact that all had a variable degree of ID before HSCT, they all made developmental progress, although normal development was not achieved at a median follow-up of 5 years. Hearing ability improved in some, but not in all patients. At the time of transplantation, median age was 3.6 (1.3-23.1) years. Therefore, HSCT is considered a feasible therapeutic option that may promote mental development in alpha-mannosidosis (Mynarek *et al.*, 2012).

Substrate reduction therapy

Miglustat (N-butyldeoxynojirimycin) acts as a competitive inhibitor of glucosylceramide synthase enzyme (glycosphingolipid synthesis) with additional effects as a chaperone and in calcium homeostasis. Miglustat has a wide tissue distribution, including the brain. Preclinical studies established that miglustat is able to cross the blood-brain barrier, reduce glycolipid accumulation and cellular pathology, and prolong survival in animal models. Clinical studies for CNS disease have been performed in GD, GM2-Gangliosidosis, and Niemann-Pick C (NPC) disease (Pastores, 2006). Miglustat has been approved for NPC therapy based on preclinical studies, a prospective clinical trial, and a retrospective cohort study (Pineda *et al.*, 2009).

Miglustat therapy provides stabilization of key neurological features of NPC. Recommendations for diagnosis and management of NPC have been published in 2009 (Baumgartner et al., 2009) and were reviewed in 2012 (Patterson et al., 2012).

In vivo studies have demonstrated that miglustat reduces GM2 storage in the CNS of the mouse model of Tay Sachs disease (TSD) and the drug increases life expectancy (Platt et al., 1997). We conducted a case study with miglustat in patients with infantile TSD and we could demonstrate that a high concentration of drug is achieved in the CSF of the patients. Miglustat was shown to prevent macrocephaly, however, neurological regression was not halted during a 12-month period (Bembi et al., 2006). Despite poor results using miglustat therapy for infantile and subacute TSD, a randomized, open-label controlled trial was conducted in a cohort of patients with juvenile gangliosidoses. Patients presented with muscle weakness, tremor and dysarthria, pyramidal and cerebellar signs, and psychiatric disturbances. At the end of the study, no significant clinical changes were observed (Maegawa et al., 2009).

General considerations for neuropsychological assessment in patients with LSD

Methods for assessing neurodevelopment in LSD will become increasingly important in view of monitoring children with LSD and understanding the efficacy of treatment, in particular for those disorders that are being considered for inclusion in neonatal screening programmes (Matern et al., 2013). Neurocognition in LSD may be impaired with distinct regression or a progressive and uneven slowing-down of development. Neuropsychological evaluation is challenged because of concurrent physical disability, behavioural disturbances, and decreased attention span. In particular, hyperactivity and fidgeting, anxiety, and stereotyped motor and verbal behaviour are difficulties encountered in evaluating subjects with LSD. Testing in a familiar environment, such as at home or day care centres, is likely to improve the feasibility of psychometric testing in these patients (Martin et al., 2008).

Routine clinical praxis emphasizes the use of standard scores to obtain normal references of typical performance. However, in children with a low level of cognitive function or cognitive decline, age-equivalent scores remain crucial to obtain information on individual learning over time and to finally obtain a curve of development in order to track changes over time. Ultimately, this approach may allow one to follow developmental progress, stagnation, and loss of abilities.

Previous studies showed inadequate representation of cognitive functions in children in this population using an overall score (Wilcox, 2004). The use of age-equivalent scores was envisaged to obtain a comparison among different domains of function for each individual patient. Furthermore, in order to evaluate longitudinal function, it is encouraged to independently evaluate different abilities including cognition, fine and gross motor skills, expressive and receptive language, social and emotional skills, and adaptive behaviour by using age-equivalent scores. For this purpose, the exploitation of different domains might allow one to define changes over time in different developmental areas.

In patients with a low level of cognitive function, in addition to the age-equivalent cognitive scores, the use of Vineland Adaptive Behavior Scales is encouraged. Recently, guidelines to assess a low level of cognitive function in behaviourally-disturbed children with LSD include specific protocols for each disease and the use of age-equivalent scores on standardized tools, such as Bayley Scales of Infant Development-II (BSID)-II and Kaufman Assessment Battery for Children-II. In addition, the use of the Vineland Adaptive Behaviour Scales for age-equivalent scores is recommended to validate results by comparing the age-equivalent scores of cognitive tests with those reported by parents (Delaney et al., 2014). Patients with LSD usually have a discrepancy between motor and mental development, and at a variable age, depending on phenotype severity (severe *versus* mild), developmental age decreases over time due to the neurodegenerative course of the disease (Valstar et al., 2011). As such, developmental assessment in LSD should be aimed to delineate intra-individual developmental pattern and identify inter-individual predictors of developmental patterns.

Non-verbal learning disorders and LSD

Gaucher disease

GD is the most common LSD with a prevalence of 1 in 40,000 live births. It is caused by mutations in the glucocerebrosidase (*GBA*) gene and decreased enzyme activity. The storage of the glucocerebroside and related metabolites in the macrophages results in a multisystem disease with stunted growth, progressive splenomegaly, anaemia, thrombocytopenia, bone pain, and skeletal anomalies. Based on central nervous system (CNS) involvement, three GD types are distinguished. GD-II and III are referred to as 'acute' and 'chronic' neuropathic GD, respectively. GD-II is characterized by acute neurodegeneration, opisthotonus and bulbar signs, and early lethality. In GD-III, a progressive neurological disease may develop at variable age with ataxia, oculomotor apraxia and horizontal supranuclear palsy, epilepsy, and behavioural disturbances. In GD type I, the chronic non-neuropathic form, the CNS is usually spared. However, GD-I patients have an increased prevalence of polyneuropathy compared with the general population (Grabowski, 2008). Also, patients with GD, even heterozygous carriers of glucocerebrosidase mutations, have been reported to be associated with an increased risk of developing Parkinson disease and Lewy Body Dementia. It is suggested that mutated glucocerebrosidase might enhance fibrillization and aggregation of alpha-synuclein protein that is necessary for formation of Lewy bodies (Chetrit et al., 2013).

In GD type III, and to a less extent in GD type I, cognitive deficits typically affect non-verbal cognition with a relative preservation of verbal skills. A comprehensive evaluation of 25 children with GD-III included neuropsychological assessment with IQ evaluation by Wechsler scales. Based on patient history examination, 19 patients had developmental delay. Full scale IQ (FSIQ) ranged from 39 to 124 (mean: 75) and about 60 per cent had below-average intellectual skills (FSIQ < 80). A significant discrepancy (> 11 points) between verbal (VIQ) and performance (PIQ) functions, reflecting a disparity in cognitive pattern, was observed in almost half of the patients, particularly in those with average or above-average IQ. In particular, specific weaknesses in perceptual organization skills, visuo-spatial reasoning, and processing speed were observed, while verbal strengths were better preserved. Patients with myoclonic epilepsy had a more severe course with distinct cognitive regression, particularly involving performance functions. There were no significant effects of the age at initiation of ERT and length of ERT on each of the IQ scores (Goker-Alpan et al., 2003; 2008).

A large cohort study conducted in eight European centres and involving 84 adult patients with non-neuropathic GD-I aimed to assess cognitive function by the CDR system, a computerised cognitive assessment system. The validated CDR composite scores used were: power of attention, continuity of attention, quality of episodic memory, quality of working memory, speed of memory, and variability of attention (Wesnes, 2006). Among the studied domains, GD-I patients scored less than age-matched healthy controls in power of attention and speed of memory, reflecting a weaker ability to focus attention and to retrieve information from both working memory and episodic memory (Biegstraaten *et al.*, 2012). However, GD-I patients did not complain of any impairment in daily activities and the clinical significance of these findings remains unknown (Elstein *et al.*, 2005).

The cause of the neuronopathic involvement in GD is still unknown. Neuropathological studies show a significant glucosylceramide storage and neuronal loss and/or astrogliosis in the hippocampal CA2-4 areas, cerebral cortical layers 3 and 5, and layer 4b of the calcarine cortex (Wong *et al.*, 2004).

Brain white matter abnormalities in children with GD were recently investigated using diffusion tensor imaging. A significant decrease of fractional anisotropy (FA) and increase of mean diffusivity parameters were observed in the cerebellar peduncles of patients with GD-III which is consistent with ataxia in these subjects. Furthermore, scattered, small lesions of white matter were observed in the whole brain of both GD-III and GD-I patients, reflecting perivascular astrogliosis. Such findings are consistent with observed variable defects in the areas of visual-spatial functions and processing speed that might reflect subcortical connectivity involvement (Davies *et al.*, 2011).

Cystinosis

Cystinosis is an autosomal recessive disorder due to mutations in the lysosomal membrane cystine transport gene, *CTNS*. It is characterized by accumulation of cystine within lysosomes. Patients present with progressive renal tubular reabsorption defect (renal Fanconi syndrome) in the first year of life and require renal transplantation by the end of the first decade. Cysteamine, used as a cystine-depleting agent, was shown to delay renal disease for many years. Despite normal intellectual functioning, cystinosis patients at all ages have a specific neuropsychological profile due to difficulties in visual-spatial and visual-motor processing and memory, and preserved visuoperceptual skills. As a consequence, children with cystinosis may be at risk of learning difficulties (Spilkin *et al.*, 2007; Besouw *et al.*, 2010). Visuo-spatial impairment was demonstrated even in very young children, treated early with cysteamine (Trauner *et al.*, 2007). Therefore, it was suggested that cystine storage *in utero*, or the effect of *CTNS* gene mutation itself, might impair myelination via oxidative stress and affect the development of cortico-cortical projections required for visuo-spatial cognition (Back *et al.*, 1998). Neuropathological studies support this hypothesis, as cystine crystals accumulate preferentially within oligodendroglial cells and their precursors. Also, microstructural changes of developing white matter were demonstrated by abnormal average diffusion properties along the dorsal visual pattern. A decrease in visuo-spatial performance was associated with reduced fractional anisotropy in the right inferior parietal lobule (Bava *et al.*, 2010).

Pompe disease

Pompe disease (also known as glycogen storage disease type II) is a progressive neuromuscular lysosomal storage disease due to the deficiency of acid alpha-glucosidase enzyme. It is characterized by accumulation of glycogen in muscle tissue, with progressive damage to respiratory, cardiac, and skeletal muscle function. Clinical presentation is variable in terms of age at onset and disease severity. Classic infantile Pompe disease presents before 1 year of age with muscle weakness and hypotonia, cardiomyopathy, and often premature death. In late-onset Pompe disease, progressive muscle weakness is the most prominent manifestation, while cardiomyopathy is observed less frequently (Kishnani *et al.*, 2013). ERT is effective and increases survival in cross-reactive immunological material (CRIM)-positive patients. CRIM-negative patients showed a limited response to ERT (Rohrbach *et al.*, 2010; Angelini *et al.*, 2012). Also, a potential limitation is that the drug cannot cross the blood-brain barrier. Neuropathological findings in infantile Pompe disease indicated neuronal loss, gliosis, and glycogen storage in the grey matter of the spinal cord, brainstem, and brain and cerebellar cortex, as well as in oligodendrocytes, and delayed myelination (DeRuisseau *et al.*, 2009). MR studies in infants may reveal bilateral symmetric deep brain white matter changes and delayed myelination (Lee *et al.*, 1996).

A systematic study of mental development was conducted in children with Pompe disease, younger than 30 months, using the Bayley Scale of Infant Development (BSID-II) during ERT. Assessment was performed after a mean duration of treatment of 15.2 months (range: 3.2-25.2) (Skriner *et al.*, 2004). Improvement in raw scores of BSID-II from baseline was documented for all patients suggesting an amelioration in cognition, language, and social abilities. However, normalized standard scores of mental performance (BSID-II mental development index; MDI) showed that these children were not functioning at exactly the same level as age-matched peers who developed normally. It was suggested that progress in the acquisition of new skills can be effectively monitored by evaluating changes in raw scores and mental performance age equivalents in children with infantile Pompe disease.

Long-term survivors treated with ERT and tested at school age scored between the low-normal range and mild developmental delay. During long-term follow-up, despite gross motor and speech developmental delay, cognitive levels were reported in the low-normal range. It was observed that assessment of cognitive function at younger age in these patients may be influenced by motor impairment (Ebbink *et al.*, 2012). More data are needed to evaluate whether longer survival by ERT unmasks the CNS phenotype in infantile Pompe disease. Adaptive functioning, measured by means of the Vineland Adaptive Behavior Scales, showed a lower adaptive level with respect to full scale IQ, probably related to motor weakness and impaired motor functions (Spiridigliozzi *et al.*, 2012).

Data on quality of life (SF-36) in large cohorts of patients with late-onset Pompe disease show that these patients scored significantly lower in physical health domains of quality of life, while they scored only slightly lower than the general population on the mental health domains (Hagemans *et al.*, 2004). Recent insights into cognitive functioning of adult patients with Pompe disease include a reduced resting functional connectivity mainly in the cingulate gyrus and medial frontal cortex of the Salience Network that plays a role in executive abilities and abstract reasoning. Accordingly, patients had significant impairment of executive functions, as measured by the Wisconsin Card Sorting test, whereas other cognitive domains were within mean normal ranges (Borroni *et al.*, 2013).

Verbal learning disorders and LSD

Neuronal ceroid lipofuscinosis

The neuronal ceroid lipofuscinosis (NCL) are a group of inherited disorders characterized by loss of motor and mental functions, epilepsy, visual loss, and premature death. An increased rate of apoptosis leading to neuronal loss and altered authophagy are key mechanisms of neurodegeneration. To date, 10 genetic loci (CLN1-10) have been identified corresponding to individual NCL types. CLN1 to 3 are the most frequent forms, corresponding to the infantile, late-infantile, and juvenile types, respectively (Bennett & Rakheja, 2013). Laboratory diagnosis is obtained by measurement in leukocytes of the lysosomal enzymes: palmitoyl-protein thioesterase (PPT) and tripeptidyl peptidase 1 (TPP1), whose mutations are responsible for CLN1 and CLN2, respectively. Molecular analyses is routinely available for CLN1, CLN2, and CLN3. Sequencing of other NCL genes may be required to establish a diagnosis (Mink et al., 2013). Neuropathological findings are indicative of diffuse cortical and cerebellar atrophy. Lysosomal storage occurs in cortical and subcortical neurons, particularly in the hyppocampal/enthorineal cortex. Ultramicroscopy shows accumulation of lipofuscin-like materials in neuronal and extraneuronal tissues. Distinct storage products may be demonstrated by electron microscopy in different tissues as granular osmiophilic dense (GROD) bodies in CLN1, the presence of curvilinear storage material in CLN2, and characteristic fingerprint inclusion bodies in CLN3 (Goebel & Müller, 2013). MRI shows cerebral and cerebellar atrophy, callosal thinning, and signal changes in subcortical nuclei. Brain analyses of cortical thickness in late-infantile NCL showed a maximum degree of reduction in the isthmus of the cingulated gyrus, thus demonstrating a differential change in cortical degeneration in this disease (Dyke et al., 2014).

Distinct neuropsychological and behavioural profiles have been depicted in patients with CLN3 (Batten/Spielmeyer-Vogt-Sjogren disease) that are characterized by a relentless course, with motor and cognitive dysfunction from school age. Visual impairment followed by seizures, extrapyramidal symptoms, sleep disturbances, and psychiatric symptoms are hallmark clinical features. A characteristic EEG finding during photic stimulation below 3 Hz is the presence of high-amplitude polyphasic spikes in the occipital region corresponding to giant visual-evoked potentials (Fig. 1). Children with CLN3 usually maintain contact with their surroundings into the second decade of life and they exhibit a characteristic compulsive speech pattern progressing to dysarthria. In the moderate stages of the disease, significant impairment is found in domains of verbal intellectual function, attention and working memory, expressive language, motor speed and dexterity, and short-term memory (Lamminranta et al., 2001). Interestingly, a particular impairment in auditory attention and memory and verbal fluency was demonstrated. This is important as these children rely on auditory abilities due to visual loss. Longitudinal observation showed retained performance on the simple auditory attention component of digit span (digits forward). In contrast, reverse digit span, with greater demands on working memory and mental manipulation of stimuli, did decline (Adams et al., 2007). Psychiatric symptoms in NCL include anxiety, aggressive behaviour, and psychotic disturbance, such as visual hallucinations, delusions, and restlessness. Aggressive behaviour manifests as low frustration tolerance and rapid changes of mood. Some behavioural features appear to reflect mental impairment in these patients. Symptoms may not be included in a specific category as each patient shows a combination of different disturbances reflecting the extent of brain pathology in CLN. A systematic study of behavioural problems in Finnish CLN3 patients, aged 9-21 years, was conducted using the Child Behavior Checklist (CBCL), Teacher Report Form (TRF), and Children's Depression Inventory (CDI). The mean total problem T-score and the mean internalizing T-score were at the borderline or clinical range, while the mean externalizing T-score was lower. Also, a significant difference in total problem T-score was recorded between females and males; the former had more severe symptoms based on both CBCL and TRF questionnaires. A minority of patients reported significant depressive symptoms on the CDI. Almost half of the patients underwent treatment with several psychotropic drugs, including citalopram and risperidone, in addition to antiepileptic drugs (Bäckman et al., 2005).

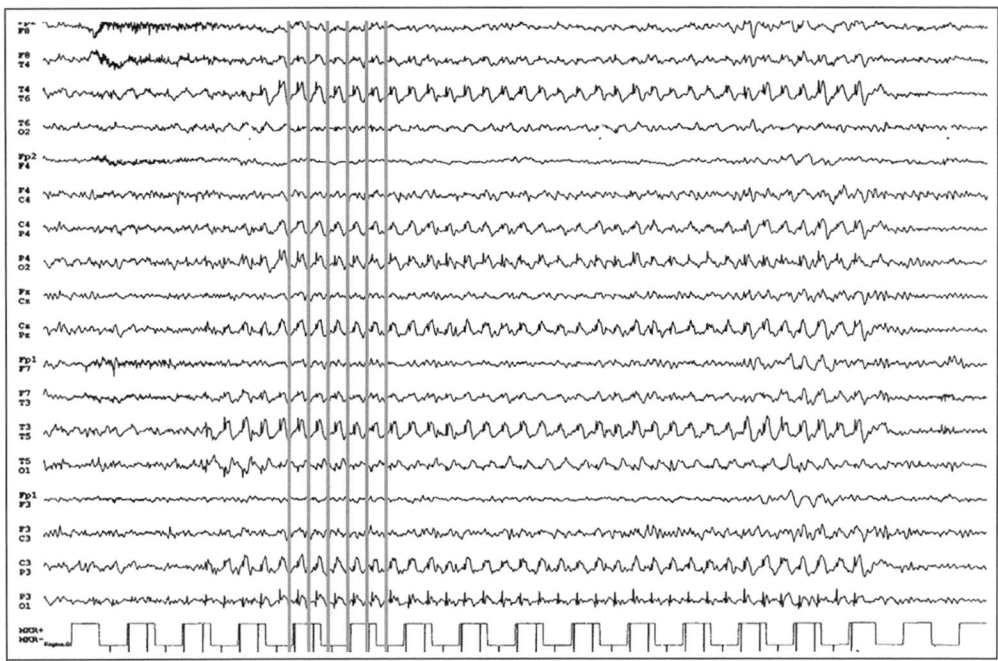

Fig. 1. EEG with photic-induced burst of high-amplitude polyphasic spike and wave activity at 3 Hz in a patient with juvenile NCL (courtesy Prof. V. Sofia, Clinic of Neurology, University of Catania).

Neuropsychological profiles and behavioural disturbances in other LSD

Mucopolysaccharidoses

The MPS are chronic and progressive multisystemic diseases caused by the storage of undegraded glycosaminoglycans (GAG) (mucopolysaccharides). Based on the enzyme defects, MPS are classified as MPS I, II, III, IV, VI and VII. GAG accumulate in the lysosomes of a wide range of tissues, resulting in a progressive and devastating multisystem disorder. MPS are diagnosed by demonstrating increased urinary GAG excretion, enzyme deficiency in leukocytes and/or fibroblasts, and by genetic analyses. Patients usually present with coarse facial features and a variable degree of skeletal anomalies known as 'dysostosis multiplex' and internal organ involvement. Progressive clouding of the cornea, heart valve disease, and hernias are other common clinical signs in these patients. Physical impairment may impact learning and development in all MPS types. CNS disease in MPS is variable and includes intellectual disability of variable degree (MPS IH, MPS II, MPS III, MPS VII), hearing loss, reduced visual acuity, hydrocephalus, seizures, and compressive myelopathy. The main neuroimaging features of MPS include global and progressive brain atrophy, hydrocephalus, abnormal white matter signals, multiple enlarged perivascular spaces, thickened meninges, and cervical cord compression (Barone *et al.*, 2002; Gabrielli *et al.*, 2004; Palmucci *et al.*, 2013; Sganzerla *et al.*, 2014). White matter lesions in MPS disorders are related to disease duration, while MRI and MR spectroscopy findings did not correlate with residual enzyme activity and urinary GAG excretion (Vedolin *et al.*, 2007a). In patients with MPS I with normal intellectual levels, decrease of white matter and reduction of corpus callosum volume on quantitative MRI analyses appear to be related to defects in attention tasks (King *et al.*, 2014).

A systematic literature review of behavioural phenotypes of the mucopolysacchiaride storage disorders indicated the occurrence of sleep disturbance and fearfulness in people with MPS I (Cross & Hare, 2013). Among all, MPS II and III behave as neurodegenerative disorders with prominent behavioural disturbances. During the first years of life, MPS II and III patients are hyperactive and impulsive children. As toddlers, they may appear prone to dangerous behaviour, often leading to body injuries. MPS II and III children have severe sleeping defects and may exhibit temper tantrums, increased irritability, and mood changes (Cross & Hare, 2013). Moreover, the MPS IIIA mouse displays hyperactivity, rapid exploratory behaviour, and has a reduced sense of danger. By analogy, MPS IIIA children explore novel environments almost continuously, disregard danger, and empathize/socialize and comply less with parents. This behavioural phenotype is reminiscent of patients with Klüver-Bucy syndrome, a condition associated with loss of amygdala function. Amygdala loss correlates with reduced fearfulness. A subset of the children with MPS IIIA show volume loss that is greater in the amygdala than in the hippocampus (Potegal et al., 2013). In MPS III, neuroimaging correlates include cerebral atrophy and progressive white matter changes (Barone et al., 1999). Mechanisms of neuropathology of MPS include storage of undegraded or partially degraded GAG and storage of secondary toxic products, such GM2 and GM3 gangliosides. However, this mechanism cannot explain the occurrence of behavioural problems encountered only in some specific MPS types. Indeed, behavioural changes are not present in MPS I, IV and VI. MPS IH patients are generally placid, gentle, and calm, although mental deterioration may occur and progress. Recently, a correlation between chemical structures of incompletely degraded HS and behaviours of patients suffering from particular MPS types was found. In particular, it was hypothesized that particular chemical moieties occurring at the ends of incompletely degraded HS molecules may determine characteristic behavioural disturbance due to chemical reactions interfering with neuronal functions (Węgrzyn et al., 2010). It has been suggested that an inflammatory response of microglial cells exacerbates the damage of MPS III neurons in the animal model. An increased expression of genes involved in inflammatory and apoptotic mechanisms has been demonstrated in the brain of MPS III mice, supporting this hypothesis (Villani et al., 2007).

Specific developmental and behavioural patterns reported for MPS II and III will be outlined below.

Mucopolysaccharidosis type II (Hunter syndrome)

MPS II is an X-linked disorder due to iduronate sulfatase deficiency resulting in the accumulation of dermatan and heparan sulphate. Systemic manifestations of MPS include coarse facial features, skeletal anomalies and joint restriction, cardiac valve disease, and hepatosplenomegaly. Extraneurological disease manifestations are controlled by systemic ERT while this is ineffective to prevent or treat CNS involvement. Based on the occurrence of neurological involvement, severe and attenuated forms are distinguished. In the attenuated form of MPS II, there is little to no CNS involvement and patients survive into adulthood (Schwartz et al., 2007). In the classic, severe form, MPS II patients have a progressive loss of cognitive functions and early death in the second decade of life. MRI findings, including white matter lesions, hydrocephalus and brain atrophy, and an elevated myo-inositol (mIns)/creatine (Cr) ratio in the grey and white matter, correlate with cognitive impairment in patients with MPS II (Vedolin et al., 2007b).

Almost 80 per cent of MSP II patients exhibit, from the first years of life, a sleep disturbance manifesting as a difficulty to initiate or maintain sleep. Other sleep-related anomalies include a decrease of rapid eye movement sleep duration, atypical sleep stage distribution, and frequent leg movements when falling asleep. Sleep disturbances manifest with a primary CNS disease in this population. Also, the onset of cognitive decline is strongly associated in these children with hyperactive behaviour, often reported as 'high-energy behaviour' and decreased attention span. Aggressiveness reflects an age-appropriate behaviour with regards to level of cognitive function, and appears to be related to frustration concerning the decline of cognitive abilities. Additional behavioural abnormalities in MPS II include "seizure-like" behaviour that manifests as absence seizures with recurrent episodes of prolonged starring per day without electroencephalographic correlates. Retrospective analyses of neurodevelopmental profiles in children with MPS II indicated some clinical markers as early predictors of cognitive dysfunction that include sleep disturbance, increased activity, behaviour difficulties, seizure-like behaviour, perseverative chewing, and inability to achieve sphincter control. A chronic perseverative chewing behaviour appears to reflect early neurological dysfunction in children with MPS II and is not observed in MPS II patients without cognitive involvement (Holt *et al.*, 2011). Such findings highlight the importance to monitor development in children with MPS II in order to identify early on those children who might benefit from CNS-directed therapy.

Mucopolysaccharidosis type III (Sanfilippo syndrome)

Sanfilippo syndrome or MPS III includes four autosomal recessive disorders (MPS III A-D) caused by deficiency of different lysosomal enzymes required for the degradation of heparan sulphate. MPS III are the most frequent among MPS disorders with an overall prevalence of 1.5-1.9 per 100,000. This is probably underestimated because of the relatively mild physical changes. Somatic features and facial coarseness are generally mild with respect to other MPS types, and patients may have an unremarkable physical appearance in the first years of life. However, early occurrence of radiographic bone changes consistent with dysostosis multiplex, including dysplastic hip and pelvic changes, may be observed (Barone *et al.*, 2001). MPS III are neurodegenerative disorders characterized by regression of intellectual and motor abilities, behavioural problems, and dementia, with death usually in the second decade of life. Recent analyses of the developmental trajectory of MPS III showed a slowing of development from the age of 2-4 years. Patients usually reach a maximum developmental level of 3.5-4 years followed by a regression from the age 4-6 years. Developmental delay, in particular speech delay, is a common presenting feature of MPS III (Valstar *et al.*, 2011). The first abilities affected by regression include speech abilities followed by mental/cognitive functions with longer preservation of motor abilities (Meyer *et al.*, 2007).

Neuropsychiatric abnormalities have been classified according to a three-stage model by Cleary and Wraith in 1993 (Cleary & Wraith, 1993). In the first 1-3 years, patients have a developmental delay, in particular for speech abilities (first phase). Almost half of patients will never be toilet-trained. At age 3-4 (second phase), behavioural abnormalities become evident with increasingly frequent and severe temper tantrums. Patients have symptoms of anxiety with panic attacks when they are in an unfamiliar environment, as well as phobias. This is followed by hyperactivity and decreased attention span and destructiveness. During this phase, children have severe sleep disturbance with an inability to fall asleep and very frequent nocturnal waking and wandering, with personal and familial distress. Modification of Strength and Difficulties Questionnaire (SDQ) scores in a sample of Italian MPS III children at various ages are reported in Tables 1 and 2 (unpublished data; Barone *et al.*).

Table 1. Behavioural disturbances, measured as SDQ (Strength and Difficulty Questionnaire) parent ratings, in pre-school children (3-5 years) with MPS III and age-matched children with normal development (ND). Personal data, unpublished

SDQ subscore	MPS III (n = 5)	ND (n = 13)	p
Emotional symptoms	2.13 (2)	1.30 (1.18)	ns
Conduct problems	2.66 (1.15)	1.76 (1.58)	ns
Hyperactivity	6.12 (2.23)	2.60 (1.6)	0.005
Peer problems	3 (1.73)	0.76 (1.01)	ns
Prosocial difficulties	6.33 (3.21)	7.76 (1.30)	ns
Total difficulties	14.3 (2.51)	14.3 (3.09)	ns

ns: not significant.

Table 2. Behavioural disturbances, measured as SDQ (Strength and Difficulty Questionnaire) parent ratings, in pre-school children (6-11 years) with MPS III and age-matched children with normal development (ND). Personal data, unpublished

SDQ subscore	MPS III (n = 8)	ND (n = 39)	p
Emotional symptoms	2.66 (0.81)	1.66 (1.39)	0.034
Conduct problems	2.33 (2.06)	1.64 (1.45)	ns
Hyperactivity	6.66 (2.33)	2.17 (1.74)	0.0063
Peer problems	4.50 (2.34)	1.23 (1.38)	0.0209
Prosocial difficulties	5.16 (2.04)	7.56 (1.94)	ns
Total difficulties	17.5 (4.63)	14.28 (3.9)	ns

ns: not significant.

The third phase of the disease starts at around 10 years and is characterized by increasing motor difficulties due to spasticity, loss of balance, and feeding disturbances. Behavioural disturbances decline with age and motor difficulties, with most patients being wheelchair-bound as teenagers. After the initial description of the natural course of MPS III, we assessed clinical and neuro-radiological correlates in MPS III patients and found that cognitive regression runs parallel to global cerebral atrophy (Fig. 2). Also, we reported that MR changes, including delayed or abnormal myelination and cerebral cortex atrophy, may precede the onset of overt neurological symptoms (Barone et al., 1999).

Psychiatric disturbances in MPS III may respond to antipsychotic drugs, however, the response to treatment is often unpredictable. The use of low dosages and very slow drug titration is recommended. The effect of risperidone (0.125-2 mg/day) was evaluated in 12 MPS III A children over a six-month period. Amelioration of symptoms related to hyperactivity and oppositional defiant and conduct disorder was observed. No significant modification with regards to weight, prolactin and serum glucose levels, nor extrapyramidal symptoms, were recorded. Large controlled blind studies are needed to prove the effectiveness of risperidone and other antipsychotic drugs in MPS disorders (Kalkan Ucar et al., 2010). Sleep disturbance and behavioural abnormalities are the first symptoms of the disease reported by parents for 38 per cent of patients and they represent a major concern in the daily management of MPS III (Mariotti et al., 2003; Fraser et al., 2005). Changes in the circadian behaviour were observed

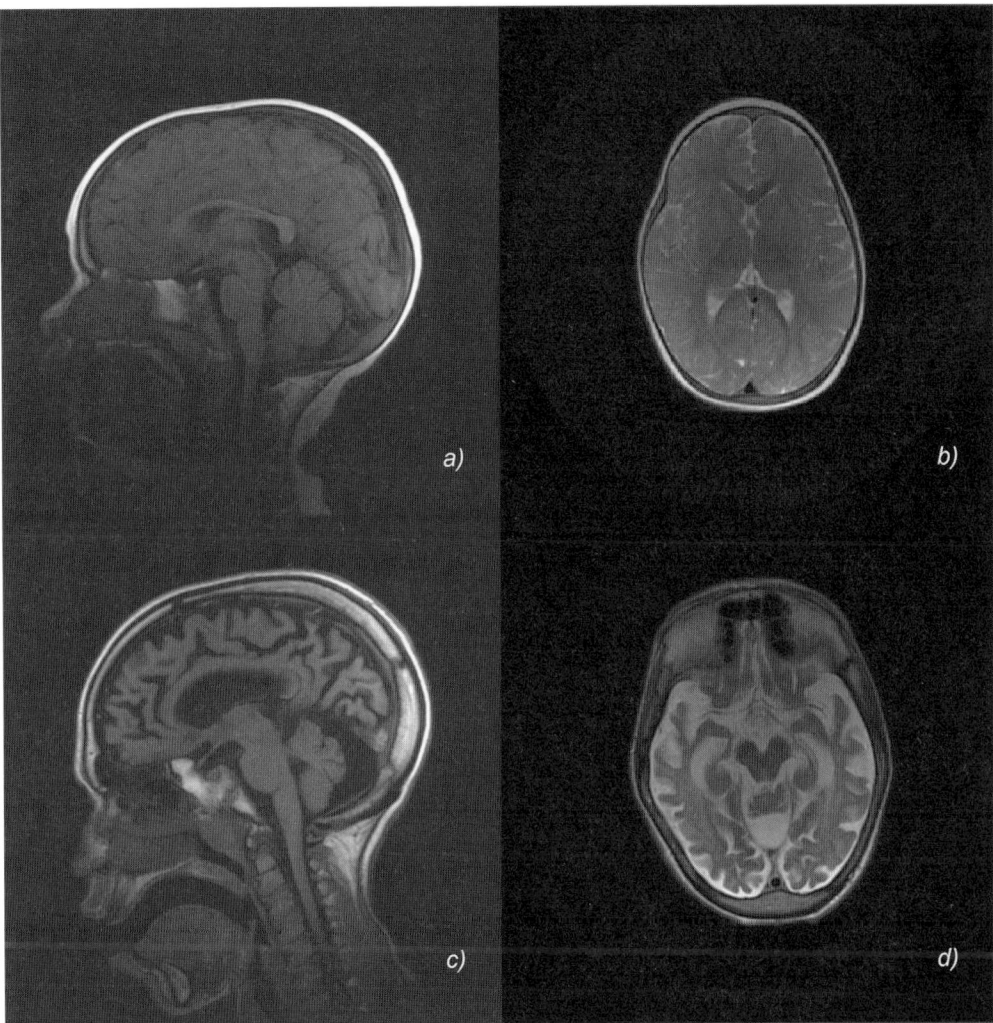

Fig. 2. Brain MR sagittal T1 and axial T2 images of Sanfilippo disease (MPS III) patients at different ages. Top (a-b): MPS III B patient, aged 17 months, with speech delay. Bottom (c-d): MPS III A patient, aged 12 years, with severe intellectual disability. Note progressive brain atrophy.

in the MPS III mice that correlate with lysosomal storage and changes in circadian neuropeptides in the suprachiasmatic nucleus which is the main biological pacemaker (Canal et al., 2010). The circadian production of melatonin is abnormal in MPS III patients and melatonin is recommended as a best-choice medication for sleep disturbance in these children (Fraser et al., 2005).

Niemann-Pick C

Niemann-Pick C (NPC) disease is an autosomal recessive disorder characterized by impaired lipid trafficking within the endo-lysosomal compartment. It is due to defective synthesis of NPC1 or NPC2 proteins and accumulation of non-esterified free cholesterol, sphingosine, sphyngolipids, and glycosphingolipids in visceral organs and the central nervous system.

Perinatal, early-infantile, late-infantile, juvenile, and adult forms are distinguished based on the age of manifestation (Patterson et al., 2012). The very early onset of NPC disease may present with foetal hydrops or neonatal cholestasis, progressive liver disease, and acute neurological deterioration. The occurrence of splenomegaly in most instances precedes the onset of neurological symptoms and may regress with age. However, splenomegaly is not mandatory for clinical diagnosis as it is absent in almost 15 per cent of patients. Neurological symptoms are also age-related and include developmental delay, clumsiness, learning difficulties, ataxia and dystonia, bulbar dysfunction, and behavioural and psychiatric disturbances. Oculomotor apraxia is a common neurological feature at all ages. The onset of neurological symptoms may be subtle and remittent, therefore masquerading the progressive nature of the disorder. In adolescence and early adulthood, neuropsychological defects in executive functions and memory may be observed (Sevin et al., 2007; Vanier, 2010).

Behavioural disturbances may appear with defective social interaction and stereotypic occupation and obsessive-compulsive behaviour in the first years as a teenager. Patients with adolescent or adult onset may present with psychotic symptoms, such as content-thought abnormality, paranoia, persecutory delusions, and visual and auditory hallucinations. Mania or depression and rapid-cycling bipolar disorder have also been described (Shulman et al., 1995; Walterfang et al., 2006). Neuroimaging studies show diffuse cerebral and/or cerebellar atrophy and white matter changes affecting the corpus callosum (Walterfang et al., 2013). Pathological studies indicate hypomyelination and axonal spheroid formation and synaptic dysfunction mainly in the Purkinje cells and in neurons of the striatum, thalamus, and hippocampus. Thus, a disruption of cortico-cortical and cortico-subcortical long tract connection and synaptodendritic changes may underpin the elevated rates of psychosis in this disorder (Pressey et al., 2012).

In NPC disease, psychotic symptoms may be resistant to standard antipsychotic treatment and mood stabilisers. Also, NPC patients may be oversensitive to motor side effects of typical neuroleptics. Specific therapy with miglustat was proven to prevent, stabilise, or partially improve neurological symptoms of NPC (Pineda et al., 2009; Di Rocco et al., 2012). Recently, clinical studies on juvenile NPC with psychiatric symptoms showed that miglustat treatment might be beneficial for reversing psychiatric features (Szakszon et al., 2014). NPC disease should be considered when subtle neurological symptoms, including swallowing or articulation difficulties, occur in young patients with psychotic symptoms or schizophrenia, in particular, when an organic mental illness and a progressive course is suspected.

Tay-Sachs disease

TSD is due to the deficiency of beta-hexosaminidase; an enzyme which leads to chronic GM2 ganglioside accumulation and progressive neurological disease. Classic TSD affects children less than 1 year old and rapidly progresses to loss of motor function, macular cherry-red spot and blindness, swallowing difficulties, and respiratory failure with early death in the first 3-4 years of life (Bley et al., 2011). Non-classic TSD includes a subacute variant with late-infantile or juvenile onset and a chronic adult form. Patients with late-onset Tay Sachs disease (LOTSD) have a more relentless clinical course with progressive mental impairment, behavioural changes, and motor deterioration with upper and lower motor neuron disease (Neudorfer et al., 2005). Neuropathological findings include neuronal ultrastructural changes with meganeurites, axonal spheroids and ectopic dendritogenesis in the thalamus, substantia nigra, cerebellum, and brainstem (Suzuki, 1991). On neuroimaging, cerebellum atrophy and global cerebral atrophy may be observed. Patients with late-onset forms may have a developmental delay with distinct regression within the first decade, including loss of language and communication, impaired socialization and repetitive behaviour, and loss of sphincter control. Gait disturbance, dystonia, and dyskinesia develop when patients grow older. In the adult form, mental abilities may be initially preserved, however, neuropsychological defects with impaired processing speed, verbal memory, and executive functions occur in up to half of the patients (Zaroff et al., 2004; Elstein et al., 2008). Schizophrenia-like features have been reported in 30 to 50 per cent of unselected patient series in adulthood. Catatonia, mania, or depression may also occur. Psychotic symptoms are resistant to neuroleptic therapy and patients are sensitive to motor side effects of typical neuroleptic medications (Neudorfer et al., 2005).

Conclusions

Development assessment and neuropsychological profiles in children with LSD contribute to define a 'behavioural phenotype' that is defined as 'a characteristic pattern of motor, cognitive, linguistic, and social abilities which is consistently associated with a biological disorder' (Flint & Yule, 1994).

Neurocognitive evaluation in children with neurodegenerative disorders, such as LSD, is a challenge because of possible, highly impaired cognitive functions and behavioural disturbances, and sensorial and physical impairments. On the other hand, accurate assessment is required in these children to monitor, early on, disease progression and outcome, particularly in view of novel therapeutic approaches for neurogenetic disorders.

Taking into account the progressive clinical course, the use of age-equivalent scores and evaluation of individual domains over time is recommended. The neurological phenotypes of LSD include some specific neuropsychological profiles and behavioural patterns underlying the dysfunction of cerebral networks. In this regard, volumetric reduction, based on quantitative MRI analyses and abnormal diffusion properties of brain white matter, have been analysed in comparison to impaired attention tasks and executive functions for several storage disorders (Vedolin et al., 2007b; Bava et al., 2010; Davies et al., 2011; Borroni et al., 2013; King et al., 2014).

LSD may result in psychiatric syndromes that may become treatment-resistant over time with disease progression. Disruptions of myelination and cortico-cortical and subcortical connectivity are common pathomechanisms for many of these disorders. Awareness of LSD can allow the clinicians to recognize disruption of neurodevelopment and secondary psychiatric illness. The knowledge of specific neuropsychological profiles and behavioural patterns in LSD may be critical for recognition, early diagnosis, and intervention programming and monitoring, and this may be helpful for families in order to plan the future care of their child (van Balkom, 2012).

Conflicts of interest: none.

References

Adams, H.R., Kwon, J., Marshall, F.J., de Blieck, E.A., Pearce, D.A. & Mink, J.W. (2007): Neuropsychological symptoms of juvenile-onset batten disease: experiences from 2 studies. *J. Child Neurol.* **22,** 621–627.

Angelini, C., Semplicini, C., Ravaglia, S., *et al.*; Italian GSDII Group (2012): Observational clinical study in juvenile-adult glycogenosis type 2 patients undergoing enzyme replacement therapy for up to 4 years. *J. Neurol.* **259,** 952–958.

Augustine, E.F. & Mink, J.W. (2013): Enzyme replacement in neuronal storage disorders in the pediatric population. *Curr. Treat. Options Neurol.* **15,** 634–651.

Back, S.A., Gan, X., Li, Y., Rosenberg, P.A. & Volpe, J.J. (1998): Maturation-dependent vulnerability of oligodendrocytes to oxidative stress-induced death caused by glutathione depletion. *J. Neurosci.* **18,** 6241–6253.

Bäckman, M.L., Santavuori, P.R., Aberg, L.E. & Aronen, E.T. (2005): Psychiatric symptoms of children and adolescents with juvenile neuronal ceroid lipofuscinosis. *J. Intellect. Disabil. Res.* **49,** 25–32.

Barone, R., Nigro, F., Triulzi, F., Musumeci, S., Fiumara, A. & Pavone, L. (1999): Clinical and neuroradiological follow-up in mucopolysaccharidosis type III (Sanfilippo syndrome). *Neuropediatrics* **30,** 270–274.

Barone, R., Fiumara, A., Villani, G.R., Di Natale, P. & Pavone, L. (2001): Extraneurologic symptoms as presenting signs of Sanfilippo disease. *Pediatr. Neurol.* **25,** 254–257.

Barone, R., Parano, E., Trifiletti, R.R., Fiumara, A. & Pavone, P. (2002): White matter changes mimicking a leukodystrophy in a patient with Mucopolysaccharidosis: characterization by MRI. *J. Neurol. Sci.* **195,** 171–175.

Baumgartner, M.R., Bembi, B., Covanis, A., et al. NP-C Guidelines Working Group (2009): Recommendations on the diagnosis and management of Niemann-Pick disease type C. *Mol. Genet. Metab.* **98,** 152–165.

Bava, S., Theilmann, R.J., Sach, M., et al. (2010): Developmental changes in cerebral white matter microstructure in a disorder of lysosomal storage. *Cortex* **46,** 206–216.

Bellettato, C.M. & Scarpa, M. (2010): Pathophysiology of neuropathic lysosomal storage disorders. *J. Inherit. Metab. Dis.* **33,** 347–362.

Bembi, B., Marchetti, F., Guerci, V.I., et al. (2006): Substrate reduction therapy in the infantile form of Tay-Sachs disease. *Neurology* **66,** 278–280.

Bennett, M.J. & Rakheja, D. (2013): The neuronal ceroid-lipofuscinoses. *Dev. Disabil. Res. Rev.* **17,** 254–259.

Besouw, M.T., Hulstijn-Dirkmaat, G.M., van der Rijken, R.E., et al. (2010): Neurocognitive functioning in school-aged cystinosis patients. *J. Inherit. Metab. Dis.* **33,** 787–793.

Biegstraaten, M., Wesnes, K.A., Luzy, C., et al. (2012): The cognitive profile of type 1 Gaucher disease patients. *J. Inherit. Metab. Dis.* **35,** 1093–1099.

Bley, A.E., Giannikopoulos, O.A., Hayden, D., Kubilus, K., Tifft, C.J. & Eichler, F.S. (2011): Natural history of infantile GM2 gangliosidosis. *Pediatrics* **128,** e1233–1241.

Borroni, B., Cotelli, M.S., Premi, E., et al. (2013): The brain in late-onset glycogenosis II: a structural and functional MRI study. *J. Inherit. Metab. Dis.* **36,** 989–995.

Calias, P., Papisov, M., Pan, J., et al. (2012): CNS penetration of intrathecal-lumbar idursulfase in the monkey, dog and mouse: implications for neurological outcomes of lysosomal storage disorder. *PLoS One* **7,** e30341.

Canal, M.M., Wilkinson, F.L., Cooper, J.D., Wraith, J.E., Wynn, R. & Bigger, B.W. (2010): Circadian rhythm and suprachiasmatic nucleus alterations in the mouse model of mucopolysaccharidosis IIIB. *Behav. Brain Res.* **209,** 212–220.

Chen, A., Dickson, P., Shapiro, E. & Harmatz, P. (2014): Intrathecal enzyme replacement for cognitive decline in mucopolysaccharidosis type I. *Mol. Genet. Metab.* **111,** S1–118.

Chetrit, E.B., Alcalay, R.N., Steiner-Birmanns, B., et al. (2013): Phenotype in patients with Gaucher disease and Parkinson disease. *Blood Cells Mol. Dis.* **50,** 218–221.

Cleary, M.A. & Wraith, J.E. (1993): Management of mucopolysaccharidosis type III. *Arch. Dis. Child.* **69,** 403–406.

Crawley, A.C., Marshall, N., Beard, H., et al. (2011): Enzyme replacement reduces neuropathology in MPS IIIA dogs. *Neurobiol. Dis.* **43,** 422–434.

Cross, E.M. & Hare, D.J. (2013): Behavioural phenotypes of the mucopolysaccharide disorders: a systematic literature review of cognitive, motor, social, linguistic and behavioural presentation in the MPS disorders. *J. Inherit. Metab. Dis.* **36,** 189–200.

Davies, E.H., Seunarine, K.K., Banks, T., Clark, C.A. & Vellodi, A. (2011): Brain white matter abnormalities in paediatric Gaucher Type I and Type III using diffusion tensor imaging. *J. Inherit. Metab. Dis.* **34,** 549–553.

De Ru, M.H., Boelens, J.J., Das, A.M., et al. (2011): Enzyme replacement therapy and/or hematopoietic stem cell transplantation at diagnosis in patients with mucopolysaccharidosis type I: results of a European consensus procedure. *Orphanet J. Rare Dis.* **10,** 6–55.

Delaney, K.A., Rudser, K.R., Yund, B.D., Whitley, C.B., Haslett, P.A. & Shapiro, E.G. (2014): Methods of neurodevelopmental assessment in children with neurodegenerative disease: Sanfilippo syndrome. *JIMD Rep.* **13,** 129–137.

DeRuisseau, L.R., Fuller, D.D., Qiu, K., et al. (2009): Neural deficits contribute to respiratory insufficiency in Pompe disease. *Proc. Natl. Acad. Sci. USA* **106,** 9419–9424.

Di Rocco, M., Dardis, A., Madeo, A., Barone, R. & Fiumara, A. (2012): Early miglustat therapy in infantile Niemann-Pick disease type C. *Pediatr. Neurol.* **47,** 40–43.

Dyke, J.P., Sondhi, D., Voss, H., et al. (2014): Differential degeneration of cortical thickness with disease progression in late infantile neuronal ceroid lipofuscinosis. *Mol. Genet. Metab.* **111,** S1–118.

Ebbink, B.J., Aarsen, F.K., van Gelder, C.M., et al. (2012): Cognitive outcome of patients with classic infantile Pompe disease receiving enzyme therapy. *Neurology* **78,** 1512–1518.

Elstein, D., Guedalia, J., Doniger, G.M., et al. (2005): Computerized cognitive testing in patients with type I Gaucher disease: effects of enzyme replacement and substrate reduction. *Genet. Med.* **7,** 124–130.

Elstein, D., Doniger, G.M., Simon, E., Korn-Lubetzki, I., Navon, R. & Zimran, A. (2008): Neurocognitive testing in late-onset Tay-Sachs disease: a pilot study. *J. Inherit. Metab. Dis.* **31,** 518–523.

Flint, J. & Yule, W. (1994): Behavioral phenotypes. In: *Child and Adolescent Psychiatry: Modern Approaches* (3rd ed.), eds. M. Rutter, E. Taylor & L. Hersov, pp. 666–687. Oxford: Blackwell Scientific Publications.

Fraser, J., Gason, A., Wraith, J. & Delatycki, M. (2005): Sleep disturbances in Sanfilippo syndrome: a parental questionnaire. *Arch. Dis. Child* **90,** 1239–1242.

Gabrielli, O., Polonara, G., Regnicolo, L., et al. (2004): Correlation between cerebral MRI abnormalities and mental retardation in patients with mucopolysaccharidoses. *Am. J. Med. Genet. A.* **125,** 224–231.

Goebel, H.H. & Müller H.D. (2013): Storage diseases: diagnostic position. *Ultrastruct. Pathol.* **37,** 19–22.

Goker-Alpan, O., Schiffmann, R., Park, J.K., Stubblefield, B.K., Tayebi, N. & Sidransky, E. (2003): Phenotypic continuum in neuronopathic Gaucher disease: an intermediate phenotype between type 2 and type 3. *J. Pediatr.* **43,** 273–276.

Goker-Alpan, O., Wiggs, E.A., Eblan, M.J., et al. (2008): Cognitive outcome in treated patients with chronic neuronopathic Gaucher disease. *J. Pediatr.* **153,** 89–94.

Grabowski, G.A. (2008): Phenotype, diagnosis, and treatment of Gaucher's disease. *Lancet* **372,** 1263–1271.

Hagemans, M.L., Janssens, A.C., Winkel, L.P., et al. (2004): Late-onset Pompe disease primarily affects quality of life in physical health domains. *Neurology* **63,** 1688–1692.

Holt, J.B., Poe, M.D. & Escolar, M.L. (2011): Natural progression of neurological disease in mucopolysaccharidosis type II. *Pediatrics* **127,** e1258–1265.

Kalkan Ucar, S., Ozbaran, B., Demiral, N., Yuncu, Z., Erermis, S. & Coker, M. (2010): Clinical overview of children with mucopolysaccharidosis type III A and effect of Risperidone treatment on children and their mothers psychological status. *Brain Dev.* **32,** 156–161.

King, K., Rudser, K., Kovac, V., et al. (2014): Attention and corpus callosum volumes in individuals with Hurler and Hurler-Scheie syndromes and controls. *Mol. Genet. Metab.* **111,** S1–S118.

Kishnani, P.S., Amartino, H.M., Lindberg, C., Miller, T.M., Wilson, A. & Keutzer, J.; Pompe Registry Boards of Advisors. (2013): Timing of diagnosis of patients with Pompe disease: data from the Pompe registry. *Am. J. Med. Genet. A.* **161,** 431–443.

Klein, A.D. & Futerman, A.H. (2013): Lysosomal storage disorders: old diseases, present and future challenges. *Pediatr. Endocrinol. Rev.* **11,** S59–63.

Lamminranta, S., Aberg, L.E., Autti, T., et al. (2001): Neuropsychological test battery in the follow-up of patients with juvenile neuronal ceroid lipofuscinosis. *J. Intellect. Disabil. Res.* **45,** 8–17.

Lee, C.C., Chen, C.Y., Chou, T.Y., Chen, F.H., Lee, C.C. & Zimmerman, R.A. (1996): Cerebral MR manifestations of Pompe disease in an infant. *AJNR Am. J. Neuroradiol.* **17,** 321–322.

Maegawa, G.H., Banwell, B.L., Blaser, S., et al. (2009): Substrate reduction therapy in juvenile GM2 gangliosidosis. *Mol. Genet. Metab.* **98,** 215–224.

Mariotti, P., Della Marca, G., Iuvone, L., Vernacotola, S., Ricci, R. & Mennuni, G.F. (2003): Sleep disorders in Sanfilippo syndrome: a polygraphic study. *Clin. Electroencephal.* **34,** 18–22.

Martin, H.R., Poe, M.D., Reinhartsen, D., et al. (2008): Methods for assessing neurodevelopment in lysosomal storage diseases and related disorders: a multidisciplinary perspective. *Acta Paediatr. Suppl.* **97,** 69–75.

Matern, D., Oglesbee, D. & Tortorelli, S. (2013): Newborn screening for lysosomal storage disorders and other neuronopathic conditions. *Dev. Disabil. Res. Rev.* **17,** 247–253.

Meyer, A., Kossow, K., Gal, A., et al. (2007): Scoring evaluation of the natural course of mucopolysaccharidosis type IIIA (Sanfilippo syndrome type A). *Pediatrics* **120,** e1255–1261.

Mink, J.W., Augustine, E.F., Adams, H.R., Marshall, F.J. & Kwon, J.M. (2013): Classification and natural history of the neuronal ceroid lipofuscinoses. *J. Child Neurol.* **28,** 1101–1105.

Mynarek, M., Tolar, J., Albert, M.H., et al. (2012): Allogeneic hematopoietic SCT for alpha-mannosidosis: an analysis of 17 patients. *Bone Marrow Transplant.* **473,** 52–59.

Neudorfer, O., Pastores, G.M., Zeng, B.J., Gianutsos, J., Zaroff, C.M. & Kolodny, E.H. (2005): Late-onset Tay-Sachs disease: phenotypic characterization and genotypic correlations in 21 affected patients. *Genet. Med.* **7,** 119–123.

Ortolano, S., Vieitez, I., Navarro, C. & Spuch, C. (2014): Treatment of lysosomal storage diseases: recent patents and future strategies. *Recent Pat. Endocr. Metab. Immune Drug Discov.* **8,** 9–25.

Palmucci, S., Attinà, G., Lanza, M.L., *et al.* (2013): Imaging findings of mucopolysaccharidoses: a pictorial review. *Insights Imaging* **4,** 443–459.

Pastores, G.M. (2006): Miglustat: substrate reduction therapy for lysosomal storage disorders associated with primary central nervous system involvement. *Recent Pat. CNS Drug Discov.* **1,** 77–82.

Patterson, M.C., Hendriksz, C.J., Walterfang, M., Sedel, F., Vanier, M.T. & Wijburg, F. NP-C Guidelines Working Group. (2012): recommendations for the diagnosis and management of Niemann-Pick disease type C: an update. *Mol. Genet. Metab.* **106,** 330–344.

Pineda, M., Wraith, J.E., Mengel, E., *et al.* (2009): Miglustat in patients with Niemann-Pick disease Type C (NP-C): a multicenter observational retrospective cohort study. *Mol. Genet. Metab.* **98,** 243–249.

Platt, F.M., Neises, G.R., Reinkensmeier, G., Townsend, M.J., Perry, V.H., Proia, R.L., Winchester, B., Dwek, R.A. & Butters, T.D. (1997): Prevention of lysosomal storage in Tay-Sachs mice treated with N-butyldeoxynojirimycin. *Science* **276,** 428–431.

Potegal, M., Yund, B., Rudser, K., *et al.* (2013): Mucopolysaccharidosis Type IIIA presents as a variant of Klüver-Bucy syndrome. *J. Clin. Exp. Neuropsychol.* **135,** 608–616.

Prada, C.E. & Grabowski, G.A. (2013): Neuronopathic lysosomal storage diseases: clinical and pathologic findings. *Dev. Disabil. Res. Rev.* **17,** 226–246.

Pressey, S.N., Smith, D.A., Wong, A.M., Platt, F.M. & Cooper, J.D. (2012): Early glial activation, synaptic changes and axonal pathology in the thalamocortical system of Niemann-Pick type C1 mice. *Neurobiol. Dis.* **45,** 1086–1100.

Rohrbach, M., Klein, A., Köhli-Wiesner, A., *et al.* (2010): CRIM-negative infantile Pompe disease: 42-month treatment outcome. *J. Inherit. Metab. Dis.* **33,** 751–757.

Schwartz, I., Ribeiro, M., Mota, J., Toralles, M.B., Correia, P. & Horovitz, D. (2007): A clinical study of 77 patients with mucopolysaccharidosis type II. *Acta Paediatr. Suppl.* **96,** 63–70.

Settembre, C., Fraldi, A., Medina, D.L. & Ballabio, A. (2013): Signals from the lysosome: a control centre for cellular clearance and energy metabolism. *Nat. Rev. Mol. Cell. Biol.* **14,** 283–296.

Sevin, M., Lesca, G., Baumann, N., *et al.* (2007): The adult form of Niemann-Pick disease type C. *Brain* **130,** 120–133.

Sganzerla, E.P., Giussani, C., Grimaldi, M., *et al.* (2014): Craniovertebral junction pathological features and their management in the mucopolysaccharidoses. *Adv. Tech. Stand Neurosurg.* **40,** 313–331.

Shulman, L.M., David N.J. & Weiner, W.J. (1995): Psychosis as the initial manifestation of adult-onset Niemann-Pick disease type C. *Neurology* **45,** 1739–1743.

Skriner, A., Corzo, D. & Kishnani, P. (2004): Mental development in patients with infantile onset Pompe Disease (IOPD) treated with enzyme replacement therapy (ERT). *Am. Coll. Med. Genet. Ann. Clin. Genet. Meeting.*

Spilkin, A.M., Ballantyne, A.O., Babchuck, L.R. & Trauner, D.A. (2007): Non-verbal deficits in young children with a genetic metabolic disorder: WPPSI-III performance in cystinosis. *Am. J. Med. Genet. B Neuropsychiatr. Genet.* **144,** 444–447.

Spiridigliozzi, G.A., Heller, J.H. & Kishnani, P.S. (2012): Cognitive and adaptive functioning of children with infantile Pompe disease treated with enzyme replacement therapy: long-term follow-up. *Am. J. Med. Genet. C. Semin. Med. Genet.* **15,** 22–29.

Suzuki, K. (1991): Neuropathology of late onset gangliosidoses. A review. *Dev. Neurosci.* **13,** 205–210.

Szakszon, K., Szegedi, I., Magyar, A., *et al.* (2014): Complete recovery from psychosis upon miglustat treatment in a juvenile Niemann-Pick C patient. *Eur. J. Paediatr. Neurol.* **18,** 75–78.

Trauner, D.A., Spilkin, A.M., Williams, J. & Babchuck, L. (2007): Specific cognitive deficits in young children with cystinosis: evidence for an early effect of the cystinosin gene on neural function. *J. Pediatr.* **151,** 192–196.

Valstar, M.J., Marchal, J.P., Grootenhuis, M., Colland, V. & Wijburg, F.A. (2011): Cognitive development in patients with Mucopolysaccharidosis type III (Sanfilippo syndrome). *Orphanet J. Rare Dis.* **6,** 43–51.

Van Balkom, I. (2012): Phenotypes and epidemiology of rare neurodevelopmental disorders. Dissertation, University of Groningen. 978-90-367-5317-3.

van Karnebeek, C.D. & Stockler, S. (2012): Treatable inborn errors of metabolism causing intellectual disability: a systematic literature review. *Mol. Genet. Metab.* **105,** 368–381.

Vanier, M.T. (2010): Niemann-Pick disease type C. *Orphanet J. Rare Dis.* **5,** 16–24.

Vedolin, L., Schwartz, I.V., Komlos, M., *et al.* (2007a): Brain MRI in mucopolysaccharidosis: effect of aging and correlation with biochemical findings. *Neurology* **69,** 917–924.

Vedolin, L., Schwartz, I.V., Komlos, M., *et al.* (2007b): Correlation of MR imaging and MR spectroscopy findings with cognitive impairment in mucopolysaccharidosis II. *AJNR Am. J. Neuroradiol.* **28,** 1029–1033.

Villani, G.R., Gargiulo, N., Faraonio, R., *et al.* (2007): Cytokines, neurotrophins, and oxidative stress in brain disease from mucopolysaccharidosis IIIB. *J. Neurosci. Res.* **85,** 612–622.

Vite, C.H., Nestrasil, I., Mlikotic, A., *et al.* (2013): Features of brain MRI in dogs with treated and untreated mucopolysaccharidosis type I. *Comp. Med.* **63,** 163–173.

Walterfang, M., Fietz, M., Fahey, M., *et al.* (2006): The neuropsychiatry of Niemann-Pick type C disease in adulthood. *J. Neuropsychiatry Clin. Neurosci.* **18,** 158–170.

Walterfang, M., Patenaude, B., Abel, L.A., *et al.* (2013): Subcortical volumetric reductions in adult Niemann-Pick disease type C: a cross-sectional study. *AJNR Am. J. Neuroradiol.* **34,** 1334–1340.

Węgrzyn, G., Jakóbkiewicz-Banecka, J., Narajczyk, M., *et al.* (2010): Why are behaviors of children suffering from various neuronopathic types of mucopolysaccharidoses different? *Med. Hypotheses* **75,** 605–609.

Wesnes, K.A. (2006): Cognitive function testing: the case for standardization and automation. *J. Br. Menopause Soc.* **12,** 158–163.

Wilcox, W.R. (2004): Lysosomal storage disorders: the need for better pediatric recognition and comprehensive care. *J. Pediatr.* **144,** S3-14.

Wong, K., Sidransky, E., Verma, A., *et al.* (2004): Neuropathology provides clues to the pathophysiology of Gaucher disease. *Mol. Genet. Metab.* **82,** 192–207.

Zaroff, C.M., Neudorfer, O., Morrison, C., Pastores, G.M., Rubin, H. & Kolodny, E.H. (2004): Neuropsychological assessment of patients with late onset GM2 gangliosidosis. *Neurology* **62,** 2283–2286.

Chapter 18

Cognitive impairment in paediatric multiple sclerosis

Angelo Ghezzi

*Neurology Operative Unit 2, Centro Studi Sclerosi Multipla, Azienda Ospedaliera S. Antonio Abate,
via Pastori 4, 21013 Gallarate, Italy*
angelo.ghezzi@aogallarate.it

Summary

Multiple sclerosis (MS) typically occurs in adults, but in 3 per cent to 10 per cent of cases it can develop before 18 years of age. Cognitive impairment (CI) has been demonstrated in all disease stages and in all clinical subtypes of MS, even at disease onset, in patients with the so-called benign course, and in subjects with paediatric onset; in these cases, CI occurs in about 30 per cent of cases, and worsens over time. Altered functions, with variable frequency, are: attention, language (receptive, verbal fluency, and naming), visual-spatial and motor functions, spatial memory, executive functions, and abstract reasoning. Fatigue and affective disorders are associated but not correlated with CI. CI is associated with limitations in social, academic, and recreational activities. Hobbies, sport activities, and quality of life are also negatively affected in patients with MS onset in childhood or adolescence. Structural damage during Central Nervous System (CNS) maturation, because of the occurrence of demyelinating lesions in pathways involved in cognition, is an important cause of CI, further limiting the acquisition of abilities. The occurrence of a *functional deficit* in addition to *structural damage* is suggested by MRI data, showing a correlation between CI and measures of brain involvement. However, compared to adults with MS, the brain is less severely and less diffusely damaged in paediatric MS, with a greater capability to compensate damage.

General aspects

Multiple sclerosis (MS) typically occurs in adults, at about 30 years, but in 3 per cent to 10 per cent of cases it can develop before 18 years of age (Banwell *et al.*, 2007).
The clinical features of paediatric MS (ped-MS) have been delineated in many retrospective and in some prospective studies; overall, they do not differ greatly from those of adult MS (A-MS), but some findings appear to be specific to ped-MS:
– onset with cerebellar and brainstem dysfunction (Banwell *et al.*, 2007; Ruggieri *et al.*, 2004), especially in children;
– polysymptomatic presentation, with fever, headache, lethargy, meningism, and seizures (ADEM-like onset), especially in very young patients (Banwell *et al.*, 2007; Ruggieri *et al.*, 2004);

– evolution with a high relapse rate, resulting in an annualized relapse rate greater than that observed in A-MS (Ghezzi, 2004; Gorman *et al.*, 2009; Renoux *et al.*, 2007; Boiko *et al.*, 2002; Simone *et al.*, 2002; Ghezzi *et al.*, 2002), at least in the initial phases of the disease;
– predominant evolution with a relapsing-remitting (RR) course, in more than 90 per cent of cases (Banwell *et al.*, 2007).

The progression of MS is slower in the paediatric population, taking a longer time to reach the level of mild (EDSS score of 3-4) and severe disability (EDSS score of 6), although this occurs at a younger age, compared to A-MS (Renoux *et al.*, 2007; Boiko *et al.*, 2002; Simone *et al.*, 2002). So far, at a given age, patients with onset in childhood are more disabled than those with a later onset.

The frequency of relapses (or the inter-attack interval) in the first few years after disease onset is a negative prognostic factor as it correlates with an increased disease severity and with an earlier entry into the secondary progressive phase of MS (Banwell *et al.*, 2007). This finding suggests that probably the inflammatory process is more pronounced in children with MS compared to adults.

Recent studies have demonstrated that cognitive dysfunction occurs in patients with ped-MS; the most relevant findings related to this topic will be reviewed in this chapter.

Cognitive dysfunction

CI is relatively frequent in A-MS as it occurs in about 40-70 per cent of cases (for a review see Chiaravallotti & DeLuca, 2008). CI has been demonstrated in all disease stages and in all clinical subtypes of MS, even at disease onset and in patients with the so-called benign course.

Various aspects of cognitive functioning are involved, including attention, information processing efficiency, executive functioning, processing speed, and long-term memory (Chiaravallotti & DeLuca, 2008). Processing speed and visual learning and memory appear to be particularly affected in MS, in more than 50 per cent of cases.

As the onset of MS typically occurs between the ages of 20 and 40 years, when individuals are most active and productive in many aspects of their lives, the occurrence of CI has an expected and demonstrated impact on daily living, household tasks, and social and vocational activities.

In the past decade, some relatively recent studies have addressed the assessment of CI in ped-MS, improving our knowledge of this topic (Chiaravallotti & DeLuca, 2008). Overall, these studies have shown that CI can be detected in more than 30 per cent of cases, and worsen over time.

The first cohort systematically investigated with a neuropsychological battery included ten children with MS (Banwell & Anderson, 2005). Tests were administered to evaluate general intelligence, receptive and expressive language, attention, visual memory, academic functioning, and executive functioning. All children failed in at least one test and some of them showed deficits in most or all cognitive areas. The deficit was more severe in children who were younger at MS diagnosis and had a longer disease duration. The severity of MS was low, suggesting that CI is independent of physical disability.

In another study (MacAllister *et al.*, 2005), attention, language, memory, and visual-spatial and motor functions were tested in a cohort of 37 patients with a mean of 14.8 years and a mean EDSS of 1.5. A total of 13 patients (35 per cent) showed CI, defined by impaired performance in at least two tests. Using the less restrictive criterion of failure of only one test, 22 patients showed mild CI (59 per cent). Attention was impaired in 30 per cent of subjects and language was also frequently affected, with impairment in naming in 19 per cent of cases and poor receptive language in 13.5 per cent; delayed recall was impaired in 19 per cent of patients. Affective disorders were diagnosed in six patients. CI correlated to EDSS, the number of relapses, age at onset, and disease length.

The occurrence of CI in ped-MS was further investigated in a large cohort of 63 ped-MS patients, who were compared with 57 demographically matched healthy controls (Amato et al., 2008). The following cognitive areas were tested: global cognitive functioning (IQ), verbal learning and delayed recall, visuo-spatial learning and delayed recall, sustained attention, abstract reasoning, expressive language, and receptive language. Five patients with MS onset before 10 years (8 per cent) exhibited an IQ of less than 70, and 17 (28 per cent) scored between 70 and 89. Criteria for significant CI (failure in at least three tests) were fulfilled in 19 patients, whereas 32 patients (53 per cent) failed at least two tests. CI was correlated with IQ level, but was independent of age, gender, relapses in the previous 1 and 2 years, EDSS, fatigue, and depression. IQ was correlated with age at onset.

In a recent study, 187 subjects with ped-MS and 44 subjects with clinically isolated syndrome were included with a mean of 14.8+2.6 years of age and a mean disease duration of 1.9+2.2 years (Julian et al., 2013). A total of 65 (35 per cent) children with multiple sclerosis and eight (18 per cent) with clinically isolated syndrome met criteria for cognitive impairment, confirming the frequency of previous studies. The areas more frequently involved were fine motor coordination (54 per cent), visuo-motor integration (50 per cent), and speeded information processing (35 per cent). The deficit was correlated with overall neurological disability.

Studies in A-MS have shown that CI worsens over time. This finding has also been confirmed in children:

– 12 ped-MS cases were re-tested 11-30 months after the basal assessment (mean: 21.6; SD: 9.3) by McAllister and colleagues (2007); the frequency at which patients performed in the impaired range increased in several tasks, with the Trail Making Test showing the largest increase in impairment frequency. An association was found between the number of tests failed and baseline EDSS; the association was slight and not significant, with the occurrence of relapses.

– Of 63 ped-MS patients of the Italian cohort, 56 were re-examined about 2 years after the first assessment (Amato et al., 2010). The entire disease duration was 5.3±3.7 years, and the mean EDSS score was 1.7±1.0. In spite of the short interval after the initial assessment, the short disease duration, and a low level of physical disability, the percentage of cases with significant CI increased to 70 per cent (Fig. 1). Thirteen patients (22.6 per cent) showed a mild cognitive impairment, and only four patients (7 per cent) remained cognitively preserved at the end of follow-up. However, after an additional follow-up of 3 years (and after 5 years from the initial evaluation), some subjects recovered and CI was finally confirmed in 50 per cent of cases. Surprisingly, when patients were re-tested 5 years after the first evaluation, the proportion of cases with CI reduced to about 50 per cent (Amato, in preparation).

– Twenty-eight patients with ped-MS and 26 age-matched controls were re-tested with a comprehensive neuropsychological battery over a 1-year period (Till et al., 2013). Seven of 28 patients (25 per cent) showed cognitive deterioration compared with only one of 26 controls (3.8 per cent); attention, processing speed, visuo-motor integration, verbal fluency, visual memory, and calculation and spelling ability were most responsive to deterioration in functioning over time. Longer disease duration was associated with greater deterioration in visuo-motor integration. Increased lesion volume was associated with slower psychomotor speed over time.

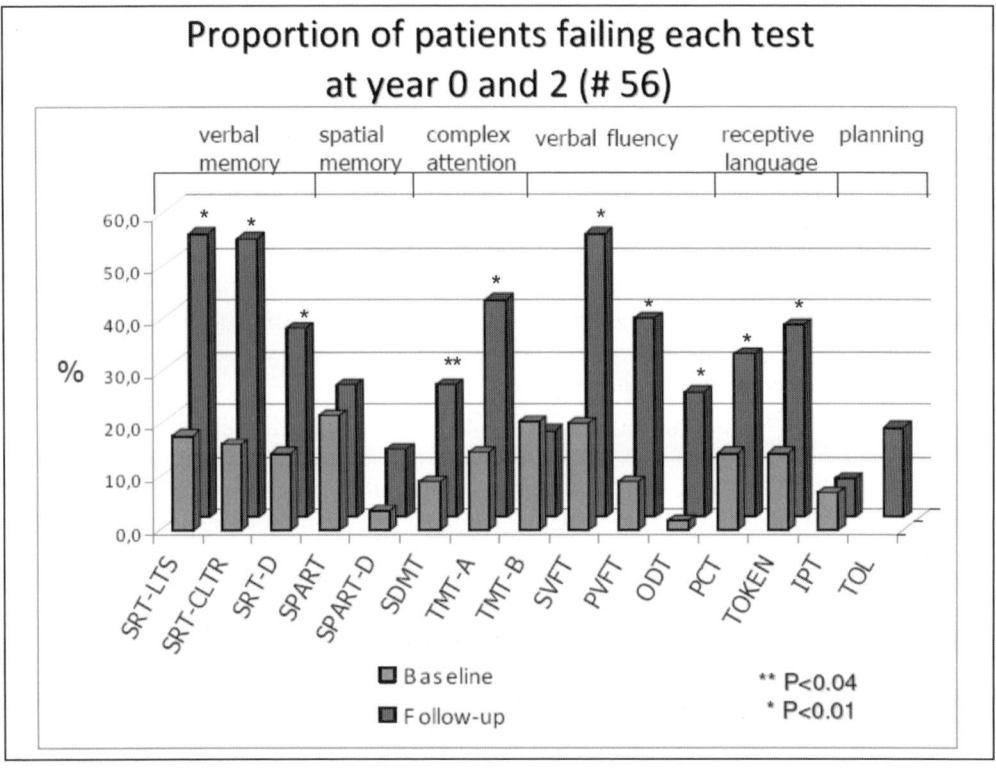

Fig. 1. Frequency and type of test failed by patients with paediatric MS at baseline and after 2 years of follow-up, according to Amato et al. (2010).

Neuropsychological batteries

Various neuropsychological batteries have been used across studies; in the future, it will be advisable to adopt a standardized battery for clinical studies as well as for screening in the clinical setting.

In the Italian study, the following neuropsychological aspects were evaluated:

– Global cognitive functioning (IQ) through the Wechsler Intelligence Scale for Children-Revised13.
– Verbal learning and delayed recall through the Selective Reminding Test and Selective Reminding Test-Delayed from the Rao Brief Repeatable Battery (BRB).
– Visuo-spatial learning and delayed recall through the Spatial Recall Test and Spatial Recall Test-Delayed from the BRB.
– Sustained attention and concentration through the Symbol Digit Modalities Test from the BRB14 and the Trail Making Tests A and B.
– Abstract reasoning through the Modified Card Sorting Test.

– Expressive language using Semantic18 and Phonemic Verbal Fluency Test19 and an Oral Denomination Test from the Aachener Aphasia Test.
– Receptive language through the Token Test, the Indication of Pictures from the Neuropsychological Examination for Aphasia, and Phrase Comprehension Test from the Battery for the Analysis of Aphasic Deficits.22.

The Pediatric Multiple Sclerosis Centers of Excellence used a comprehensive network battery consisting of 11 tests, addressing the following cognitive domains:
– general ability level: Wechsler Abbreviated Scale of Intelligence-2 subtest battery 11 including Vocabulary and Matrix Reasoning subtests;
– reading and language: Wechsler Individual Achievement Test II Pseudoword Decoding, Expressive One Word Picture Vocabulary Test, and the Wechsler Abbreviated Scale of Intelligence Vocabulary subtest;
– attention, working memory, and speeded processing: Digit Span test from the Wechsler Adult Intelligence Scale IV (for 16 years of age and above) or the Wechsler Intelligence Scale for Children IV (for younger than 16 years of age), Wechsler Adult Intelligence Scale, or Wechsler Intelligence Scale for Children coding test;
– executive functioning: Contingency Naming Test, Delis Kaplan Executive Function System Trail Making Test;
– verbal episodic learning and recall: California Verbal Learning Test-Child version or II (as appropriate for age);
– visuo-spatial functioning: Beery-Buktenica Developmental Test of Visual-Motor Integration-sixth edition 18 and the Wechsler Abbreviated Scale of Intelligence Matrix Reasoning;
– fine motor speed and coordination: Grooved Pegboard Test 19 and Delis Kaplan Executive Function System Trail Making Test-Motor Speed Condition.

In a recent consensus paper, addressing the design of clinical trials in ped-MS, cognitive functioning was included among the measures of clinical outcome (Chitnis et al., 2013). The following domains are considered relevant in clinical evaluation, and also applicable to very young subjects (the suggested test is provided in brackets):
– attention (Symbol Digit Modalities Test, Trail Making Test A);
– executive functioning (Trail Making Test B, CNT);
– verbal learning and memory (Spatial Recall Test);
– visual-spatial processing, learning, and memory (Beery Visual-Motor Integration, BVMTR);
– language (D-KEFS fluencies, WASI vocabulary);
– general intelligence (WASI or WISC-IV).

Given the frequency of CI and its impact on daily activities and school/social performances, there is a common need for sensitive and feasible screening tools. Starting from a comprehensive neuropsychological battery, an attempt has been made to identify the tests which most effectively discriminate against CI (Portaccio et al., 2009); the selective Reminding Test, the Symbol Digit Modalities Test, the Trail Making test, and the Vocabulary Reminding test from the Wechsler Intelligence Scale for Children yielded a sensitivity of 96 per cent and a specificity of 76 per cent, and were suggested as tools for a brief neuropsychological battery for children.

Psychosocial issues

The most relevant issues are summarized in Table 1. CI is associated with limitations in social, academic, and recreational activities. MS-related school absences and assistance with school activities have been reported in 10 per cent to 35 per cent of cases (MacAllister et al., 2005;

Amato *et al.*, 2008; Banwell *et al.*, 2007). School difficulties were more prominent for subjects with lower social status and poorer housing conditions (Mikaeloff *et al.*, 2010). Some patients had to repeat school due to school absences or cognitive difficulties; hobbies and sport activities were also negatively affected and this was observed in 34 per cent of the Italian cohort (Amato *et al.*, 2008).

Fatigue and affective disorders can coexist with CI and contribute to the impairment of social activities. Affective disorders were diagnosed in 6 of 13 children who underwent a structured psychiatric evaluation (major depression and anxiety disorder, not otherwise specified, in two; major depression in two; anxiety, not otherwise specified, in one; and panic disorder and generalized anxiety disorder in one) (Banwell & Anderson, 2005). The rate of depression was lower in the Italian cohort (6 per cent); data were further analyzed including the Kiddie-SADS-Lifetime Version-PL semi-structured interview, showing an increased frequency of cases with affective disorders; major depression was found in 15 per cent, depression and anxiety in 5 per cent, panic disorders in 5 per cent, and bipolar disorders in 5 per cent of 39 children (Amato *et al.*, 2008; MacAllister *et al.*, 2009).

Fatigue was found in 9 of 63 cases with a cut-off score of 4 in Fatigue Severity Scale, as proposed for adults, but in 46 (73 per cent) using a cut-off score of 2, corresponding to the fifth percentile of healthy controls (Amato *et al.*, 2008). Behavioural changes were reported by parents in 39 per cent cases of the Italian cohort (Amato *et al.*, 2008; MacAllister *et al.*, 2009).

Table 1. Frequency of psychological, social, and cognitive issues involved in paediatric MS patients (Banwell & Anderson, 2005; MacAllister *et al.*, 2005; Amato *et al.*, 2008; Julian *et al.*, 2013; McAllister *et al.*, 2007; Amato *et al.*, 2010; Till *et al.*, 2013)

Emotional disorders	6%-46%
Behaviour abnormalities	Around 40%
Fatigue	30%-73%
Difficulties at school	Around 30%
Reduced hobbies and sport activities	34%
Cognitive impairment	Severe: around 30% Mild: > 50% Increasing with time

Fatigue and quality of life have been recently investigated in a study including 51 ped-MS patients, who were examined with self- and parent-report scales (Goretti *et al.*, 2010). Fatigue was assessed by means of the PedsQL Multidimensional Fatigue Scale that includes scales to measure fatigue, sleep disturbances, and cognitive fatigue; quality of life was assessed via the pedsQL scales, providing measures of physical, emotional, social, and school functioning. EDSS was the only variable associated with fatigue and QoL. Fatigue correlated with sleep difficulties, cognitive problems, and QoL variables (Goretti *et al.*, 2012).

Neuroimaging and pathophysiology of cognitive impairment

CI in A-MS has been variably correlated with many patterns of brain damage, as measured by MRI; lesion volume, brain atrophy, thalamus atrophy, grey-matter lesions, and normal-appearing white matter involvement. Other studies have addressed the pattern of brain activation in preserved/cognitive impaired patients, and relation to cognitive tasks, by means of functional MRI (Chiaravallotti & DeLuca, 2008).

Information provided by these studies can only partially be extrapolated from ped-MS as the mechanisms involved in brain damage and recovery in a developing brain are different to that of A-MS patients; ped-MS patients are more likely develop lesions in the posterior fossa, and T2 lesions more frequently disappear during follow-up (Chabas *et al.*, 2008; Waubant *et al.*, 2009; Fields, 2008). Using non-conventional techniques, it has been observed that in ped-MS patients, normal-appearing-white-matter (NAWM) is more preserved and grey matter (GM) is less involved (Tortorella *et al.*, 2006).

The correlation between neuropsychological function and brain MRI measures has been addressed in a study including 35 ped-MS patients and 33 age- and sex-matched healthy controls (Till *et al.*, 2011). Thalamic volume, total brain volume, and grey matter volume were lower in MS patients compared to control, moreover, patients with CI and those without CI were distinguished based on corpus callosum area and thalamic volume. Thalamic volume accounted for significant incremental variance in predicting global IQ, processing speed, and expressive vocabulary, and was the most robust MRI predictor of cognition relative to other MRI metrics.

The key role of thalamus involvement in ped-MS has been demonstrated in another study, showing significant bilateral grey matter loss in the thalamus, significantly correlated with T2 LL, with sparing of the cortex and other deep GM nuclei (Mesaros *et al.*, 2008; Rocca *et al.*, 2009).

Ped-MS patients studied by means of functional MRI showed an increased recruitment of the left primary sensorimotor cortex and a reduced functional connectivity between the left primary sensorimotor cortex and the left thalamus, the left insula and the left secondary sensorimotor cortex, the supplementary motor area and the left secondary sensorimotor cortex, the left thalamus and the left insula, and the left thalamus and the left secondary sensorimotor cortex. The interesting finding was that activation of brain areas was more restricted compared to adult RR and SP MS patients (Rocca *et al.*, 2014). These findings have been interpreted as the structural background that accounts for the more favourable clinical outcome at short term in ped-MS. The progressive recruitment of cortical networks over time in adult RR patients might result in a loss of their plastic reservoir contributing to subsequent disease progression. The more pronounced brain plasticity in ped-MS probably also accounts for the partial recovery of CI at long term, after a severe short-term decline.

Because of the crucial role of myelin in optimizing mechanisms of learning and information processing (Till *et al.*, 2011), demyelinating lesions during CNS maturation in pathways involved in cognition are an important structural cause that account for CI in ped-MS patients. As impairment of visuo-spatial memory, attention, executive functions, and language strongly involve cognitive and academic performances, activities such as listening to lengthy instructions, organization of unstructured assignments, generation of novel ideas, efficient processing speed, and organization of cognitive and behavioural strategies are likely compromised (Banwell & Anderson, 2005). In other words, cognitive dysfunction during biological and psychological development is likely to involve an impairment of cognitive structures necessary for future acquisitions of academic achievements and cognitive strategies; the combination of structural damage plus a functional deficit may explain the severe drop of CI in the short term, however, given the more pronounced plasticity of the brain, the brain has the capability to recover and partially compensate the deficit (Fig. 2).

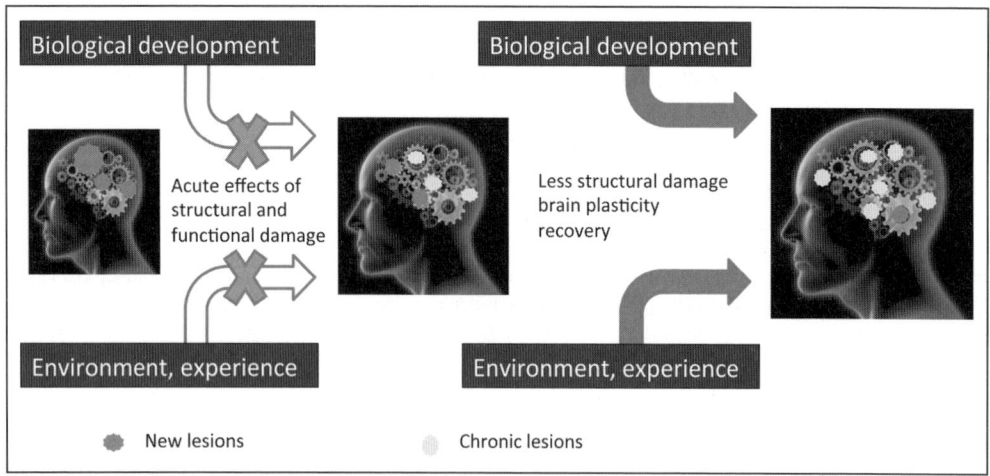

Fig. 2. Possible mechanisms involved in the development of cognitive impairment in the paediatric MS population, and mechanism limiting its evolution during follow-up.

Conclusions

To summarize, CI occurs in a high proportion of cases with ped-MS, increasing in frequency and severity after a short-term follow-up. Altered functions, with variable frequency, are: attention, language (receptive, verbal fluency, and naming), visual-spatial and motor functions, spatial memory, executive functions, and abstract reasoning (Banwell & Anderson, 2005; MacAllister et al., 2005, 2007; Amato et al., 2008, 2010; Julian et al., 2013; Till et al., 2013). Fatigue and affective disorders are associated, but not correlated, with CI.

Structural damage during CNS maturation in pathways involved in cognition is an important cause of CI, further limiting the acquisition of abilities. The occurrence of a *functional deficit* in addition to *structural damage* is suggested by MRI data, showing that brain damage is less severe and the capability to compensate damage is greater in paediatric than in adult MS patients. This finding is also suggested by clinical studies showing that ped-MS have less severe physical impairment compared to A-MS with a similar disease duration, as ped-MS patients reach moderate or severe disability after a longer interval, about 10 years later (Renoux et al., 2007). It is possible that children and adolescents activate compensatory mechanisms limiting the extent of CI during the long-term evolution of the disease (Fig. 2). To verify this issue, it will be important to have long-term data on cognitive functioning of ped-MS patients (Portaccio et al., 2010).

At present, no valid therapeutic strategies are available; symptomatic treatment in A-MS has not demonstrated any positive effect, whereas some positive results have been observed in response to immune-active drugs (Amato et al., 2013), in particular to natalizumab (Iaffaldano et al., 2012). Cognitive rehabilitation could be effective, but this field must be better explored by further studies.

Conflicts of interest: none.

References

Amato, M., Goretti, B., Ghezzi, A., et al.; Multiple Sclerosis Study Group of the Italian Neurological Society. (2008): Cognitive and psychosocial features of childhood and juvenile MS. *Neurology* **70**, 1891–1897.

Amato, M., Goretti, B., Ghezzi, A., et al.; Multiple Sclerosis Study Group of the Italian Neurological Society. (2010): Cognitive and psychosocial features in childhood and juvenile MS: a reappraisal after two years. *Neurology* **75**, 1134–1140.

Amato, M.P., Langdon, D., Montalban, X., et al. (2013): Treatment of cognitive impairment in multiple sclerosis: position paper. *J. Neurol.* **6**, 1452–68.

Banwell, B.L. & Anderson, P.E. (2005): The cognitive burden of multiple sclerosis in children. *Neurology* **64**, 891–894.

Banwell, B., Ghezzi, A., Bar-Or, A., Mikaeloff, Y. & Tardieu, M. (2007): Multiple sclerosis in children: clinical diagnosis, therapeutic strategies, and future directions. *Lancet Neurol.* **6**, 887–902.

Banwell, B., Krupp, L., Kennedy, J., et al. (2007): Clinical features and viral serologies in children with multiple sclerosis: a multinational observational study. *Lancet Neurol.* **6**, 773–781.

Boiko, A., Vorobeychik, G., Paty, D., Devonshire, V. & Sadovnick, D; University of British Columbia MS Clinic Neurologists. (2002): Early-onset multiple sclerosis: a longitudinal study. *Neurology* **59**, 1006–1010.

Chabas, D., Castillo-Trivino, T., Mowry, E.M., Strober, J.B., Glenn, O.A. & Waubant, E. (2008): Vanishing MS T2-bright lesions before puberty: a distinct MRI phenotype? *Neurology* **7**, 1090–1093.

Chiaravalloti, N.D. & DeLuca, J. (2008): Cognitive impairment in multiple sclerosis. *Lancet Neurol.* **7**, 1139–1151.

Chitnis, T., Tardieu, M. & Amato, M.P; International Pediatric MS Study Group Clinical Trials Summit: meeting report. (2013). *Neurology* **80**, 1161–1168.

Fields, R.D. (2008): White matter in learning, cognition and psychiatric disorders. *Trends Neurosci.* **31**, 361–370.

Ghezzi, A. (2004): Clinical characteristics of multiple sclerosis with early onset. *Neurol. Sci.* **25**, S336–339.

Ghezzi, A., Pozzilli, C., Liguori, M., et al. (2002): Prospective study of multiple sclerosis with early onset. *Mult. Scler.* **8**, 115–118.

Goretti, B., Ghezzi, A. & Portaccio, E. (2010): Psychosocial issue in children and adolescents with Multiple Sclerosis. *Neurol. Sci.* **31**, 467–470.

Goretti, B., Portaccio, E., Ghezzi, A., et al.; Multiple Sclerosis Study Group of the Italian Neurological Society. (2012): Fatigue and its relationships with cognitive functioning and depression in paediatric multiple sclerosis. Multiple Sclerosis Study Group of the Italian Neurological Society. *Mult. Scler.* **18**, 329–334.

Gorman, M.P., Healy, B.C., Polgar-Turcsanyi, M. & Chitnis, T. (2009): Increased relapse rate in pediatric-onset compared with adult-onset multiple sclerosis. *Arch. Neurol.* **66**, 54–59.

Iaffaldano, P., Viterbo, R.G., Paolicelli, D., et al. (2012): Impact of natalizumab on cognitive performances and fatigue in relapsing multiple sclerosis: a prospective, open-label, two years observational study. *PLoS One* **7**, e35843.

Julian, L., Serafin, D., Charvet, L., et al.; Network of Pediatric MS Centers of Excellence. (2013): Cognitive impairment occurs in children and adolescents with multiple sclerosis: results from a united states network. *J. Child Neurol.* **28**, 102–107.

MacAllister, W.S., Belman, A.L., Milazzo, M., et al. (2005): Cognitive functioning in children and adolescents with multiple sclerosis. *Neurology* **64**, 1422–1425.

MacAllister, W.S., Christodoulou, C., Milazzo, M. & Krupp, L. (2007): Longitudinal neuropsychological assessment in pediatric multiple sclerosis. *Dev. Neuropsych.* **32**, 625–644.

MacAllister, W.S., Christodoulou, C., Troxell, R., et al. (2009): Fatigue and quality of life in pediatric multiple sclerosis. *Mult. Scler.* **15**, 1502–1508.

Mikaeloff, Y., Caridade, G., Billard, C., Bouyer, J. & Tardieu, M. (2010): School performance in a cohort of children with CNS inflammatory demyelination. *Eur. J. Paediatr. Neurol.* **14**, 418–424.

Mesaros, S., Rocca, M.A., Absinta, M., et al. (2008): Evidence of thalamic gray matter loss in pediatric multiple sclerosis. *Neurology* **70**, 1107–1112.

Portaccio, E., Goretti, B., Lori, S., et al.; Multiple Sclerosis Study Group of the Italian Neurological Society. (2009): A brief neuropsychological battery for children: a screening tool for cognitive impairment in childhood and juvenile multiple sclerosis. *Mult. Scler.* **15**, 620–626.

Portaccio, E., Goretti, B., Zipoli, V., et al. (2010): Cognitive rehabilitation in children and adolescents with multiple sclerosis. *Neurol. Sci.* **31**, S275–278.

Ruggieri, M., Iannetti, P., Polizzi, A., Pavone, L. & Grimaldi, L.M; Italian Society of Paediatric Neurology Study Group on Childhood Multiple Sclerosis. (2004): Multiple sclerosis in children under 10 years of age. *Neurol. Sci.* **25**, S326–335.

Renoux, C., Vukusic, S., Mikaeloff, Y., *et al.*; Adult Neurology Departments KIDMUS Study Group. (2207): Natural history of multiple sclerosis with childhood onset. *N. Engl. J. Med.* **365,** 2603–2613.

Rocca, M.A., Absinta, M., Ghezzi, A., Moiola, L., Comi, G. & Filippi, M. (2009): Is a preserved functional reserve a mechanism limiting clinical impairment in pediatric MS patients? *Hum. Brain Mapp.* **30,** 2844–2851.

Rocca, M.A., Valsasina, P., Absinta, M., *et al.* (2014): Intranetwork and internetwork functional connectivity abnormalities in pediatric multiple sclerosis. *Hum. Brain Mapp.* **35,** 4180–4192.

Simone, I.L., Carrara, D., Tortorella, C., *et al.* (2002): Course and prognosis in early-onset MS: comparison with adult-onset forms. *Neurology* **59,** 1922–1928.

Tortorella, P., Rocca, M.A., Mezzapesa, D.M., *et al.* (2006): MRI quantification of gray and white matter damage in patients with early-onset multiple sclerosis. *J. Neurol.* **253,** 903–907.

Till, C., Ghassemi, R., Aubert-Broche, B., *et al.* (2011): MRI correlates of cognitive impairment in childhood-onset multiple sclerosis. *Neuropsychology* **3,** 319–332.

Till, C., Racine, N., Araujo, D., *et al.* (2013): Changes in cognitive performance over a one-year period in children and adolescents with multiple sclerosis. *Neuropsychology* **27,** 210–219.

Waubant, E., Chabas, D., Okuda, D.T., *et al.* (2009): Difference in disease burden and activity in pediatric patients on brain magnetic resonance imaging at time of multiple sclerosis onset *vs.* adults. *Arch. Neurol.* **66,** 967–971.

Mariani Foundation
Paediatric Neurology Series

1: Occipital Seizures and Epilepsies in Children
Edited by: *F. Andermann, A. Beaumanoir, L. Mira, J. Roger and C.A. Tassinari*

2: Motor Development in Children
Edited by: *E. Fedrizzi, G. Avanzini and P. Crenna*

3: Continuous Spikes and Waves during Slow Sleep – Electrical Status Epilepticus during Slow Sleep
Edited by: *A. Beaumanoir, M. Bureau, T. Deonna, L. Mira and C.A. Tassinari*

4: Metabolic Encephalopathies: Therapy and Prognosis
Edited by: *S. Di Donato, R. Parini and G. Uziel*

5: Neuromuscular Diseases during Development
Edited by: *F. Cornelio, G. Lanzi and E. Fedrizzi*

6: Falls in Epileptic and Non-Epileptic Seizures during Childhood
Edited by: *A. Beaumanoir, F. Andermann, G. Avanzini and L. Mira*

7: Abnormal Cortical Development and Epilepsy – From Basic to Clinical Science
Edited by: *R. Spreafico, G. Avanzini and F. Andermann*

8: Limbic Seizures in Children
Edited by: *G. Avanzini, A. Beaumanoir and L. Mira*

9: Localization of Brain Lesions and Developmental Functions
Edited by: *D. Riva and A. Benton*

10: Immune-Mediated Disorders of the Central Nervous System in Children
Edited by: *L. Angelini, M. Bardare and A. Martini*

11: Frontal Lobe Seizures and Epilepsies in Children
Edited by: *A. Beaumanoir, F. Andermann, P. Chauvel, L. Mira and B. Zifkin*

12: Hereditary Leukoencephalopathies and Demyelinating Neuropathies in Children
Edited by: *G. Uziel, F. Taroni*

13: Neurodevelopmental Disorders: Cognitive/Behavioural Phenotypes
Edited by: *D. Riva, U. Bellugi and M.B. Denckla*

14: Autistic Spectrum Disorders
Edited by: *D. Riva and I. Rapin*